Health-care professionals and acclaimed authors celebrate Dr. Bruno Cortis' groundbreaking approach to healing the

HEART AND SOUL

"I can confirm everything Dr. Cortis says in this long-needed book about the importance of self-affirmation, self-empowerment, self-responsibility, and self-healing—not just for the heart patient, but for everyone."

—Bernard Virshup, M.D., clinical professor of
behavioral sciences, UCLA School of Medicine

"*HEART AND SOUL* is a magnificent and inspired work written by a courageous and compassionate physician who reveals the awesome power of the heart to heal. . . . This book is a historic contribution to wellness health care."

—Edward A. Taub, M.D., president,
Foundation for Health Awareness

"Dr. Cortis is a physician who is also a healer. . . . *HEART AND SOUL* speaks to our deepest needs as human beings—the need for meaning, love, and forgiveness. This book is a healing for the soul as well as for the body."

—Joan Borysenko, Ph.D., author of
Minding the Body, Mending the Mind

"I was stunned by the power of his words. . . . It will serve as a valuable tool for physicians and patients across this land."

—Joe Graedon, author of *Joe Graedon's New People's Pharmacy*

"Dr. Bruno Cortis writes from the heart—for the heart. This is a much needed and very important book."

—Gerald G. Jampolsky, M.D., coauthor of *Love Is the Answer*

"Bruno Cortis has written the book I needed but could not find when I had a heart attack. . . . Here is what you need to know about your heart and how to care for it. Dr. Cortis takes the 'victim' out of heart attack."

—Arthur Frank, author of *At the Will of the Body: Reflections on Illness*

"Faith and love, two mighty healing powers, radiate from Dr. Cortis through the pages of *HEART AND SOUL*. They will heal millions."

—Carleton Whitehead

"Dr. Cortis shares care and love with the patient as a whole person, instead of focusing narrowly on 'the disease.' HEART AND SOUL is a cri de coeur on how being of good heart is part and parcel of reaping the rewards of a good and healthy heart for both patient and physician."

—Benjamin S. Llamzon, Ph.D., author of
A Human Case for Moral Intuition

"It is splendid! It is wonderful! It is a must-read for anyone who wants to take charge of their life and their body."

—Michael C. Rann, pastor, First Church of Religious Science,
Science of Mind Center

"Society has known for thousands of years that 'heart' is not a physical organ, but is symbolically the organ most affected by love. If you really love your own heart, follow the wise advice Dr. Cortis provides."

—C. Norman Shealy, M.D., Ph.D., founding president,
American Holistic Medical Association

HEART
AND SOUL

*A Psychological and Spiritual Guide
to Preventing and Healing
Heart Disease*

BRUNO CORTIS, M.D.

POCKET BOOKS
New York   London   Toronto   Sydney   Tokyo   Singapore

POCKET BOOKS, a division of Simon & Schuster Inc.
1230 Avenue of the Americas, New York, NY 10020

Copyright © 1995 by Bruno Cortis, M.D.

Published by arrangement with Villard Books

Library of Congress Cataloging-in-Publication Data

Cortis, Bruno.
    Heart and soul : a psychological and spiritual guide to preventing and healing heart disease / Bruno Cortis.
        p.   cm.
    Previously published: New York : Villard Books, 1995.
    Includes bibliographical references and index.
    ISBN: 0-671-55140-X
    1. Heart—Diseases—Psychosomatic aspects. I. Title.
RC682.C677 1997
616.1'2—dc20   96-38556
                                                CIP

First Pocket Books trade paperback printing March 1997

10 9 8 7 6 5 4 3 2 1

POCKET and colophon are registered trademarks of Simon & Schuster Inc.

Cover design by Matt Galemmo

Printed in the U.S.A.

This book is dedicated to

Pia, Veronica, Maximillian,

my parents, Aunt Amelia,

and my patients.

Acknowledgments

This book would not have been possible without the generosity of many people who have touched my life. I want first of all to acknowledge my patients, who, through their pain, allowed me to discover their humanity and to see them as individuals. They gave me the courage to share my own humanity.

Thanks also to Carleton Whitehead, a spiritual teacher who taught me self-love, self-discovery, and to see beyond the emotions.

Thanks to Zoe Keithley, who first encouraged me to write about my life and guided me in organizing a manuscript called "Our Hearts Are the Same." Some of that material has been integrated into this book.

I thank Tom Ferguson, an exceptional writer and very inspiring friend. With Tom's guidance I worked for nearly two years; he wrote the initial outline of this book and inspired the creation of the Exceptional Heart Patients Program. Tom allowed me to discover a new dimension in writing and guided me in the process. I appreciate his help immensely.

Thanks to Michael Rann, for inspiring me to see pathways to self-realization.

I acknowledge my friends Dr. Harry Mercado, Carol Mercado, Dr. John Henry Pfifferling, Dr. Bernie Virshup, Dr. Joe Graedon, Dr. Mike Mercer, and Dr. Ben Llamzon, for reviewing the initial manuscript and for their constant support and encouragement during the progression of the book.

I have been inspired and deeply touched by the work of Dr. Gerry Jampolsky, Dr. Bernie Siegel, Dr. Herbert Benson, Dr. Joan Borysenko, Dr. Dean Ornish, and Dr. Deepak Chopra.

I acknowledge Kathryn Lance for helping me to communicate my feelings, and Jeff Herman, my agent, who supported me and created a bridge of friendship with Kathryn Lance.

I acknowledge the guidance, support, and expert editing of Emily Bestler. I acknowledge Marie Bellavia for her secretarial assistance.

I acknowledge my parents for having given me life and for educating me to love and respect others.

Special gratitude to Aunt Amelia, who showed me how to love.

I acknowledge my wife, Pia, for her love, support, and patience in many difficult times of life. I recognize her as a mother, as a wife, as a physician, and as a supportive friend.

I acknowledge my children, Veronica and Maximillian, for their constant love and for their patience during my busy professional life.

Finally, I acknowledge the people in my life who touched my heart and compelled me to touch other people's hearts.

Contents

Introduction

BEATING THE ODDS:

EXCEPTIONAL HEART

PATIENTS

Allow me to introduce myself. I am Dr. Bruno Cortis, a fifty-nine-year-old cardiologist. In this book I want to share with you what I have learned in my thirty years of medical practice. By sharing my knowledge with you, I hope to help you improve or preserve the health of your heart.

The things that I want to share extend beyond the realm of medical knowledge. They have to do with joy, with happiness, and with the spirit. They encompass the patient-physician relationship and the relationship of the patient to his or her true, innermost self. Many are lessons that I've learned not from medical school but from my patients.

I want to share these things because I believe that our inner essence is spiritual and that disease is first of all a mental and emotional event that manifests itself in the body secondarily. I believe that disease is well within the power of the patient to control and that its cure is not dependent only on high-tech medical solutions. As a physician, I no longer want to limit myself and my life to the care of the sick. I would much rather reach people who are healthy and show them how to stay well. So please read on and learn how these lessons can transform your life as they have transformed mine.

TALES OF TWO EXCEPTIONAL HEART PATIENTS

At the age of sixty-five, Dr. White, a professor of psychology, had a massive heart attack. His doctors told him he would need a quintuple-bypass operation. Dr. White's father and two brothers had died at an early age of coronary artery disease, and Dr. White, now limited to a sedentary existence, had every reason to believe that the active part of his life was over. Yet he refused to accept the doctors' gloomy prognoses. After the bypass operation and cardiac rehabilitation, Dr. White returned to work. Six years later he is still working, and his life is as full as that of a man half his age. He has done everything he wanted to, including trekking in the Himalayas.

Ben, age fifty-eight, whose family also had a history of heart disease, discovered in a diagnostic procedure that one of his coronary arteries was almost completely blocked. The test also showed that his heart had been visibly damaged. Ben submitted to a procedure known as angioplasty, which can unblock clogged arteries but does not repair previous heart damage. Just a few months after the angioplasty, tests showed that Ben's heart had become much stronger and had somehow healed itself.

Medical miracles? Definitely. Flukes? Not at all. The fact is that Dr. White and Ben are just two of hundreds of patients I know who not only have managed to beat the medical odds on heart disease by surviving it but have also gone on to resume full and meaningful lives in spite of it.

What made the difference? Why did these two men thrive

when so many patients with similar diagnoses become "cardiac cripples" or even die? I was determined to find out. I began to interview heart patients, trying to discover a common denominator in their backgrounds, lifestyles, and the medical treatment they received. The more I studied the question, the more I became convinced that their experiences had to do with something beyond these obvious factors.

Most doctors agree on the predisposing factors that contribute to heart disease, and most people today know about them. They are smoking, high blood pressure, elevated cholesterol, lack of exercise, excess weight, diabetes, genetics, and stress. But what most people don't know is that these factors are present in only 50 percent of heart patients. How can we explain the person who has a normal cholesterol level yet most of whose arteries are plugged up? Even stranger cases involve patients who have high cholesterol levels but completely clear and healthy arteries. I've seen patients in their eighties with high cholesterol. They live beautiful, healthy lives and have not suffered from heart disease.

THE THREE TYPES OF HEART PATIENTS

My research has convinced me that a patient's emotional and psychological *responses* to heart disease are often as important as or more important than the type or extent of heart disease that person happens to have. Patients tend to be divided into three groups:

• Passive patients, who typically respond to a diagnosis of heart disease with pessimism, fear, and denial.
• Obedient consumer patients, who follow the doctor's orders but do not take much personal initiative.
• Exceptional heart patients, who respond to their condition with optimism and hope.

Passive patients are unwilling to take responsibility for their condition. They blame outside forces, withdraw from their social contacts, and bewail their fate. Many become deeply depressed. They grow negative, despairing, and hopeless. They tend to die very soon after their diagnosis.

Some passive patients almost seem to welcome a diagnosis of heart disease. I sometimes feel that these patients have a conscious or unconscious death wish. They don't really want to live. They don't want to fight the disease. The bottom line is they don't want to change.

Obedient consumers are the A students of modern medicine. They follow their doctors' orders to the letter. They quickly sense what their doctors want them to do and how their doctors want them to behave, and they do so, sometimes at the cost of not verbalizing how they could contribute. They typically have average outcomes. They frequently die exactly when their doctors predict they will.

Exceptional heart patients respond in a very different way. After the initial shock of the diagnosis, exceptional heart patients come to see their heart disease as a challenge, an opportunity to deepen their knowledge and broaden their awareness. While they might well have realistic fears for the future, they make a conscious choice to respond to their situation in a proactive way, taking full responsibility. They are determined to do everything in their power to bring their lives into balance, to do all they can to understand their condition and make the maximum possible effort to recover. They develop their own personal responses to their ailing hearts.

These patients speak of their situation in words and tones that express excitement and hope. They have come to consider their new concern for their hearts as an invitation to reexamine their lives. They have looked deeply into their lives and into their hearts, and they have the courage and perseverance to make the changes required to bring their lives into balance.

TAKING YOUR HEART INTO YOUR HANDS

The powerful force of the mind in healing all kinds of diseases is being increasingly acknowledged by the scientific community. While researchers still debate the mechanisms by which positive effects are produced, hundreds of thousands of real people with real health problems are coming to the conclusion that there is a great deal more they can do in managing and healing their own illnesses than they had been led to believe. I am convinced that these exceptional patients have been successful not just because of their involvement and cooperation with medical treatments but because of the methods they have employed on their own.

Many exceptional heart patients go through a profound personal transformation. They overcome internal conflicts and make significant changes in their habits of thinking and behaving. Above all, they have discovered ways to tap into a profound will to live. And by doing so they activate a powerful biological force within themselves.

I must admit that in some ways these findings came as a surprise to me. The idea that patients can take charge of their own health and be responsible for their own healing was not something we learned in medical school. As a doctor I had been trained to look only at the disease the person had, not at the person who had the disease. I was taught that it was my job to serve as a sort of medical mechanic, making people better by giving them drugs and subjecting them to diagnostic tests and surgical procedures. I had always assumed that good patients were those who obeyed their doctors' orders.

In my interviews with heart patients, I saw a different picture. Exceptional heart patients did not always obey doctors' orders. In fact, they often caused their doctors a good deal of trouble by questioning their advice, refusing to go along with their proposed treatments, or seeking second opinions. They demanded a great deal of information about their conditions, much more than their doctors were accustomed to providing. They made use of alternative and experimental treatment methods of which their doctors knew very little. In short, they insisted on doing things their own way.

The exceptional heart patients I interviewed kept the reins of their health care in their own hands. They wanted their doctors to serve as advisers and consultants, not as authorities. They resented it if their doctors attempted to run the show. They insisted on making the final decision themselves.

Exceptional heart patients did not all show concern for their hearts in the same way. Indeed, I was struck by the extent to which each exceptional heart patient seemed to have developed a unique self-treatment plan. While there was considerable overlap, they all appeared to use a particular technique in different and sometimes conflicting ways. Even when it looked as if they had reached very similar destinations, close questioning revealed that their journeys had led them down very different paths.

As I expected, many employed some form of diet, exercise, stress management, meditation, psychological practice, spiritual involvement, and active participation with friends and family.

But, try as I might, I could discover no formula, no single set of directions for becoming an exceptional heart patient. Many of these patients surprised me by attributing their unexpected success to methods most doctors know little about; clearly expressing to their physicians their own needs; developing spiritual or psychological insights; increasing the number of conversations with friends and family members; using messages received in dreams, positive affirmations, prayer, guided visualizations, religious experiences; and being open to the power of love.

CONFOUNDING YOUR DOCTOR

Indeed, the responses of exceptional heart patients to their illness seemed so medically idiosyncratic that their doctors would commonly roll their eyes or throw up their hands as they recounted their medical histories. But there was one aspect of their histories that could not be ignored. Many of these patients confounded their doctors by getting better when they were supposed to get worse. They thrived when they were supposed to weaken. They lived when they were supposed to die.

We physicians are just beginning to appreciate a phenomenon that many people have been aware of for a long time—the vast power the mind and emotions have in helping people overcome disease. While I do not mean to imply that you can cure yourself in an afternoon merely by wishing on a star, I have been greatly impressed by the importance of hope, optimism, faith, and self-responsibility in the exceptional heart patients I have interviewed. These men and women seem to have gone through a profound process of change, a process I have come to think of as *health empowerment*. This vital transformation can make all the difference in the outcome of an illness. It can be the difference between life and death.

Doctors are taught that all patients are the same, but the fact is that patients vary enormously in their response to a diagnosis of heart disease. Some will make radical changes in the way they think and live and eat and exercise and relate to others. Others will react with defensiveness and denial and will resist even the most minor changes.

It is not my role to tell you how you should care for your heart. You have every right to be a passive patient if you wish. But if you wish instead to be an exceptional heart patient, then read on. The purpose of this book is to help you become exactly that.

Each of the exceptional heart patients you will meet here has a special perspective to offer. No two have responded to their diagnosis in the same way. Each individual has developed unique priorities and created a personalized health plan.

PATIENT-CENTERED HEALTH

I believe that the exceptional heart patients I have known are pioneers in the transition from an old, doctor-centered health-care system to a new, patient-centered one, not only for treating heart disease but for approaching every treatment of every ailment. From the old medical point of view, we were only supposed to follow doctors' orders. From the new point of view, there is so much more we can do both to prevent and to heal our diseases. From the old point of view, the things these patients have accomplished may look like miracles. However, I would suggest that in the dawn of this new health-care system, such self-directed healing and self-management of health is not a miracle at all but our birthright.

We now understand that to take care of your heart, the best thing you can do is be fully informed, fully involved, and fully responsible. Feeling powerless, feeling afraid, and feeling that you are in the dark about what is going on are actually *bad* for the heart. It is not healthy for you to feel at the mercy of your doctors. Your doctors are doing their best, but they cannot heal your heart for you. You yourself must make the decisions as to how you will handle your health. There is a wisdom inside you that has more profound healing powers than all your doctors put together.

In this book I will show you how you can learn to tap this innate power. I will explain how your heart works, and how you can keep it healthy and strong. I will address the relationship between you and your doctor, and show you how to forge that relationship into a partnership dedicated to your spiritual and physical health. I will lead you through the most important physical, psychological, and spiritual factors that combine to make a healthy heart and body. Throughout I will offer you questionnaires and quizzes that you can use to gauge your own heart health, as well as Heartskills, practical, hands-on exercises designed to have an immediate, positive impact on your heart.

So, whether you are a heart patient or merely concerned about the health of your heart, I urge you to turn the pages now and learn how other people have managed to become exceptional heart patients, and how you can too.

HEART
AND SOUL

Chapter One

YOU AND YOUR HEART

Heart attack is a misnomer. The heart never attacks you.
It is the source of your life.

—B. Cortis

*H*eart disease has changed my life. I'm not talking about my heart disease, because I have a healthy heart. I'm talking about the heart disease of my patients, especially the ones I call exceptional heart patients. Despite their illness, these men and women all have one thing in common: They enjoy life. When you see them for the first time, you don't even suspect that they have had heart problems, a heart attack, or surgery. Mr. Kurtz, a sixty-one-year-old manual laborer who is working full-time after two heart attacks, is one example. "Why should I quit working?" he asks. "Why should I quit anything? I like my work. I like walking two miles a day. I like my wife and family. I like laughter."

Patients like Mr. Kurtz have helped me to change, after thirty years as a physician, and have sent me in search of meaning and purpose in life. They have transformed my thinking about health. Thanks to these patients, I have realized that health depends on self-development and spiritual growth, and that these experiences are a result of loving others and sharing yourself with them. My patients have taught me through my daily work—crying with them when they suffer, standing aside with awe and respect when they choose to die, and rejoicing when the recovery they desire becomes a reality.

My patients have taught me many facts that I never learned in medical school. Now I want to share these lessons with you. They can save your life, keep you out of the cardiology unit, or—even better—keep you from ever developing heart problems. If you already have heart disease, these truths can empower you so that recovery becomes a miracle that leaves your whole life open to the health and happiness that you may have thought (as I once did) could only be exaggerated optimism or a dream.

THE DEADLIEST ILLNESS

If you ask people to name the deadliest common ailment, most will answer cancer or AIDS. I have known patients who were so obsessed by the idea of getting cancer that they lived their entire lives in fear. It's true that the rates of certain cancers have been rising for a generation. Likewise, AIDS is a terrifying illness that is spreading, and the world will be a far better place when researchers find a vaccine or cure for it.

But what most people don't realize is that the number-one killer in America is heart disease. By every measure—expense, pain, time lost from work, families destroyed—it is by far the most devastating common illness. Over one and a half million Americans have a heart attack each year, and one-third of them die. In fact, every thirty-four seconds another human life is lost to this killer. Forty-three percent of all Americans die of some form of cardiovascular disease. In 1991, 923,422 Americans died from heart and blood-vessel illnesses, while cancer claimed

514,300 and AIDS 29,800. The American Heart Association estimates that in 1994 the cost of cardiovascular disease will be $128 billion.

So what? you may ask. Isn't heart disease only an ailment of the elderly? Not really. In fact, more than 156,000 Americans under the age of sixty-five die of this disease every year. Forty-five percent of all fatal heart attacks strike people under sixty-five, and 5 percent strike people under forty.

Another common misconception is that, thanks to modern medicine, heart disease is no longer deadly. After all, when someone has a heart attack today, can't he or she just be cured with a bypass? Nothing could be further from the truth or more dangerous to believe. In the first place, approximately a third of all heart attacks are fatal. About 300,000 people die each year before even reaching the hospital.

In the second place, despite advanced medical and surgical techniques, modern medicine *can't really cure* heart disease. It's true that a blocked artery can often be cleaned out with an angioplasty, a procedure in which a small balloon is inflated inside the artery to flatten the blockage. But 25 to 35 percent of all clogged arteries treated with angioplasties become reblocked within six months. As for a coronary bypass, the procedure literally bypasses the problem. A section of clean vein is inserted to detour blood flow around the diseased artery. The cause of the heart disease, the reasons for the artery being clogged, remains and can recur.

YOUR HEALTH IS YOUR RESPONSIBILITY

All modern medicine can do then is apply temporary fixes. For a true cure, for a new relationship with your heart, you are your only resource. Your doctor can set the stage for healing, but only you can heal.

Unfortunately, many patients think of their heart disease as *my* problem. They come into my office carrying an invisible bag on their back. The bag is full of all the bad habits and medical problems they have ever had, such as abuse of tobacco, lack of exercise, overeating, chest pain, and breathlessness. When they enter my office, they dump the bag on my desk, look for the most comfortable chair to put themselves in, and say, "Doc, you take care of it."

In some cases I *can* take care of the problem. But in too many others I can't because the disease has gone too far or the patient refuses to change the conditions that caused it. Still, so many of these patients have an inner faith that no matter what they do to their own bodies, "Doc" will take care of it.

That's just not true. It's a dangerous illusion.

It's true that I will do everything I can to help. But I can't do it on my own. I can only do it with my patients' support and help.

That's why I want to propose a new way of looking at heart disease, one in which you become a partner with your doctor, a partner in the care and well-being of your heart. Only then can you really begin to heal. But for this new partnership to work, you must take a great deal of responsibility. The first step toward that responsibility is to learn more about that wonderful organ, your heart.

Know Your Heart

You already know that your heart is a powerful muscle that circulates your blood through your body. Each day your heart beats 100,000 times, pumping nearly 2,000 gallons of blood. Over the course of a seventy-year life span, your heart beats more than 2.5 billion times! Despite all the work it does, your heart is only about the size of a fist. It weighs about half a pound.

Though many feelings seem to fill it sometimes, it is hollow inside. The four hollow chambers of the heart fill with blood and then pump it, through one-way valves. The right side takes in used, poorly oxygenated blood in the receiving chamber (atrium) and pumps it from the second chamber (ventricle) to the lungs, where it gives up carbon dioxide and becomes freshly oxygenated. The blood then travels to the atrium on the left side of the heart, where it is pumped via the left ventricle to the rest of the body. The primary route for sending out fresh blood is the body's main artery, the aorta.

From the aorta, the blood enters the arteries that branch out from it, as if it were a tree. Each branch has branches, in descending sizes, going down to the smaller arteries, the arterioles, with thin, elastic walls that can open up or close as the body's needs dictate.

The heart also has a blood supply of its own: the two main coronary arteries and their smaller branches, which surround the heart like a crown (corona). The coronary arteries, like any arteries, can become clogged, leading to one form of heart attack.

Don't Wait for a Heart Attack

So you can see that the heart is a truly remarkable pump, continually sending life-giving blood throughout the body. But suppose you have a damaging heart attack. What then happens to its performance?

Close your hand into a fist. Now open it and extend all your fingers. Close it again. Open it and extend your fingers. Do this several more times. Get the feel of it? This rhythmic action represents the pumping action of your healthy heart. Now let's pretend you've had a mild heart attack. Continue to open and close your fist, but hold your thumb down to represent a damaged portion of heart muscle. The hand isn't quite as vigorous as before, but it still opens and closes.

Now let's pretend that you've had a second heart attack, or that the first one was more severe. Continue to open and close your hand, but hold down the index finger along with the thumb. Feel the difference? This is what happens in a severe heart attack. The loss of power makes it very difficult for the heart to do its job.

Now let's make things even more difficult. Let's suppose you also have high blood pressure. Blood pressure is the measurement of the push of the blood against the arterial walls when the heart muscle is contracted. In a healthy person, the arteries are elastic and give easily in response to the pressure. But what if the arterial walls are no longer elastic, or if the arterioles are constricted because of cold or tension instead of being wide open as they usually are? In these cases the heart has to work even harder, pumping *against* the constriction of millions of tiny narrowed arteries. This extra effort against resistance is measured as high blood pressure. As many as sixty million Americans have high blood pressure and 35 percent don't know they have it.

Now you can see the connection between the health of the heart and the circulatory system. When the arteries and arterioles are narrowed for any reason, the heart has to pump with extra effort just to do its job of supplying blood to the body. The extra workload causes an increased thickness of the heart's walls and may cause the chambers to become enlarged.

Now let's say that, in addition to this high blood pressure, you have a severe heart attack—one where you're holding down two fingers. You can see right away the disastrous consequences for the rest of your body and the health of the remainder of your heart. How is your damaged heart going to pump against all that resistance? How will the blood get around and carry its food to the body cells?

What Causes Heart Disease

Coronary artery disease can be caused by many factors. The most common, and potentially the most serious, is the narrowing of arteries caused by deposition on their walls of cholesterol and cellular debris. You can think of it as similar to the mineral buildup water can leave inside pipes. After a time such deposits, known as plaque, can narrow an artery to the point where only a trickle of blood can get through or the flow is stopped altogether. This condition is known as *atherosclerosis*, or hardening of the arteries.

Atherosclerosis is the number-one killer in the United States today. It is so deadly because a blocked artery can produce a direct assault on the heart. The amount of damage done by this assault depends on several factors.

If the blocked artery is one of the two major arteries to the heart, the situation can be very serious and even fatal. For instance, if the main left coronary artery is blocked, the whole left side of the heart will be damaged or die. If, on the other hand, a smaller branch artery is blocked, the condition is less serious.

Usually arteries become blocked when a blood clot originates in a narrowed artery. This can also cause a heart attack, or, if the clot gets stuck in an artery in the brain, a stroke.

Not every blocked artery produces a heart attack or stroke. Sometimes I see patients with an occluded artery who have never had a heart attack because their condition came on slowly. Their bodies had a chance to adjust and increase the capacity of other arteries to take up the slack for the one that was failing.

There are also other ways a heart attack occurs. Sometimes, for example, a coronary artery goes into a spasm, shutting itself off. If the spasm lasts long enough, it can cut off the blood supply to the heart as effectively as a blockage. Because such spasms can be caused by emotional stress, this kind of heart attack offers one of the clearest and most interesting proofs of the close connection between the mind and the body.

Arrhythmias, or irregular heartbeats, can cause your heart to beat less effectively. In some cases they are linked to disorganization of the heart's normal rhythm and heart attack. The two most common types of potentially fatal arrhythmias are *ventricular tachycardia*, in which the heart beats abnormally fast, and *ventricular fibrillation*, in which the synchronized beating of the heart is replaced by an uncoordinated, inefficient quivering. Both of these usually originate in a part of the heart muscle that has already been damaged. If untreated, this form of arrhythmia can lead to sudden death.

Silent Killers

So we have seen the interdependence of the heart and the circulatory system. Both must work reasonably well, and one cannot work imperfectly without affecting the other immediately.

Anything that threatens one of these systems threatens the whole body. Diabetes, with its serious sugar imbalance and propensity for forming clots, is a threat to heart and circulation. Likewise, tobacco use raises the heart rate and steals oxygen from the blood while diminishing the lungs' ability to draw in and hold oxygen. High blood pressure keeps up a merciless demand on both the heart and the arteries.

Many of the diseases that attack the heart and circulation are called silent diseases because you cannot always tell from a person's physical appearance that he or she is in trouble. Nor is age always an indicator. I have treated young people for heart attack and have examined eighty-year-olds with the hearts of twenty-year-olds.

There are, of course, some ways to predict the likelihood of heart trouble. When one or more of the risk factors are present, for example, disease is more likely. Smokers' risk of a heart attack is more than twice that of nonsmokers. Genetic predisposition to certain diseases also seems to be a factor. Diabetes, heart disease, alcoholism, and cholesterol problems are all known to run in families. Does this mean that if your father died of heart disease you are doomed? Not at all. In fact, you can benefit from this early warning sign.

HEART DISEASE AS A MESSAGE FROM YOUR BODY

I can't help thinking of a patient I saw recently. She came into the hospital in shock and was found to have septicemia, an infection in the blood. She weighs over 300 pounds, and she had obviously been very sick for a long time before she came to us for help.

We are doing everything possible for her. Antibiotics, IV fluids, medication to keep her blood pressure normal. But why in the world did she wait so long before showing up? Couldn't she have chosen a moment when she could still be treated? I remember reading somewhere that 60 percent of our lifetime medical expenses are incurred during the six months before we die. This is a measure of the intensity of service required in the last half year of life. But does it need to be that way?

I feel that most of us are like this patient. We go through life ignoring our bodies' signals, disregarding symptoms until a crisis occurs.

But the body talks to us, and it is up to us to listen and try to understand the message. This is especially true with the heart. Remember that the heart bears the load of all our physical as well as our mental and emotional activity. Stress can affect the heart just as strongly as it does any other body system. And the heart reacts just the same as any other body system.

"I'm in trouble," it may tell you. "I'm feeling overstressed. I'm not getting enough oxygen."

Just what do these messages mean?

Perhaps the most common warning of impending heart trouble is angina.

Angina pectoris, or chest pain, is the result of a reduced blood supply to the heart. This reduced supply of blood (and therefore oxygen) is also known as *ischemia*. Commonly, angina is brought on by physical activity or emotional stress, though some people have angina while at rest. This latter form of angina may be induced by a coronary spasm. Estimates are that 3,150,000 people have angina pectoris.

Angina is not always experienced as pain in the chest. Sometimes it feels like pressure or tightness in the chest, neck, arms, jaw, or upper back. Often it is accompanied by palpitation or shortness of breath.

One of my patients described her angina as "like a big cramp in my chest going completely through the back." Another patient said that it was like "a big weight on my chest."

Angina does not necessarily mean that a heart attack is imminent, but it is a sign that your heart, for some reason, is receiving an insufficient amount of blood. Unfortunately, many people shrug off angina, assuming that it is a pulled muscle or indigestion.

Another warning sign involves the major arteries of the legs. In this case the leg muscles are not getting enough oxygen, and they can painfully cramp up, often after only a few steps of walking. After rest the cramps ease. This warning sign is known as *intermittent claudication*, and it is a signal that your leg arteries are narrowed.

Arrhythmias, or irregular heartbeats, can also be signs of trouble. The most common arrhythmia is called a skipped heartbeat (it is actually a premature contraction). It feels like a palpitation or fluttering in the chest and is usually harmless. Other arrhythmias cause the heart to beat too fast (tachycardia) or too slow (bradycardia). If these conditions last long enough, they can lead to a variety of symptoms, from light-headedness and fatigue to loss of consciousness or even death. Arrhythmias can be provoked by high or low levels of certain minerals in the blood, or by use of cigarettes, alcohol, and drugs. Emotional stress can also bring on arrhythmias. While an occasional "skipped beat" may be nothing to worry about, continuing or recurrent arrhythmias are important messages from your body and should be checked out.

Sometimes your heart gives you little warning that it is in trouble. Angina and even a heart attack can be painless. It is estimated that 4 percent of the population, most of them middle-aged men, suffer from silent ischemia. Any adult with several risk factors, and especially with a family history of heart disease, should be tested for this condition.

HEARTSKILL 1: LEARNING TO TAKE YOUR OWN PULSE

One evening I was feeling the pulse of a patient. It was strong, with regular intervals, warm and vibrating with life. The thought came to my mind that I was in touch with God at that moment and that, just by feeling our pulse, we can be in touch with the very center of our lives whenever we wish.

The pulse is actually a wave of blood sent through the arteries each time the heart contracts. By measuring the pulse, we can assess the number of heartbeats per minute. Pulse rate therefore provides important information about cardiac function.

The pulse can be felt wherever an artery passes close to the skin. It can be measured at the wrist, elbow, neck, temple area, groin, behind the knee, and on top of the foot. Most commonly the wrist is used. To appreciate the pulse, place your index and middle finger over the underside of the opposite wrist. Press gently and firmly until you locate the pulse. Don't use your thumb to feel the pulse, because it has a pulse of its own, which could interfere with the true count.

Count the pulse for fifteen seconds, then multiply by 4 to get your heart rate.

HOW YOU CAN CALCULATE YOUR HEART RATE

Step   What to Do
1   Apply two fingers to your wrist and find your pulse beat.
2   Count your pulse beats for 15 seconds.
3   Multiply the number of pulse beats you found in Step 2 by 4 to find your heart rate.

NOTES: A.   Your *heart rate at rest* may vary between 60 and 100 beats per minute. The average is about 70 beats per minute.

            B.   Do this simple calculation to find your *maximum heart rate* during exercise:
Subtract your age from 220, that is,
220 − Your Age = _____.

Whenever you take your pulse, pay attention to both the rate (beats per minute) and the regularity. A regular pulse is one where there is a constant interval between beats. If you can feel that the interval between one beat and another varies under the same circumstances, then your pulse is irregular. If this seems to be a recurring condition, you should consult your doctor.

To learn what's normal for you, take your pulse several times, at different times of the day, for a week or so, and record the numbers for the following categories:

Resting pulse: The resting pulse is usually the slowest rate and should be taken in the morning after you wake up. The average rate is about 70. A slow pulse is one that beats fewer than 60 times per minute, while a rapid pulse is above 100 beats a minute at rest. Various conditions, such as depression or some drugs, can cause a slower than normal pulse. A healthy young athlete often has a very slow pulse. Likewise, a rapid pulse can have many causes, including illnesses and alcohol, tobacco, or caffeine use. If your resting pulse is consistently too fast or too slow, you should consult your doctor. Treatment usually focuses on eliminating the cause of the condition.

Postexercise pulse: During exercise the pulse rate should be kept near the *target heart rate*. You can calculate yours by using a simple formula. First, determine your maximum heart rate (the fastest rate your heart can beat) by subtracting your age from 220. The best exercise level is 50 to 75 percent of this maximum rate. This range is called your target heart rate.

For a fifty-year-old, the target range is calculated by subtracting his age from 220 (170), and then taking 50 percent and 75 percent of that figure, for a target heart range of 85 to 127 beats per minute.

Check your own postexercise heart rate immediately after finishing exercise. If you find it is higher than your target heart range, this is a message from your heart to exercise less vigorously until you are in better physical condition. If you are a regular exerciser and your rate suddenly goes up, the message is the same: Slow down.

It is also useful to know your *recovery rate*, the amount of time it takes your pulse to return to normal after exercise. To determine recovery rate, take your pulse immediately after exercise and then again each minute until your heart returns to resting rate. That amount of time is your recovery heart rate: My experience is that the heart should return to the resting rate within three to five minutes. The better conditioned you are, the faster your recovery rate will be.

Get to know your own resting pulse, exercise rate, and recovery rate. This will give you a picture of the individual way your heart works. If you are beginning an exercise program (see Chapter 10), you will probably be able to observe each of the rates becoming slower. If, however, any of the rates changes suddenly, consult your doctor.

Chapter Two

YOU AND YOUR DOCTOR

Where there is love for mankind
there is love for the art of healing.
—Hippocrates

If you're like most Americans, you take great care of your car. You wash it; you see that the tires and fluid tanks are all full. You make sure that you fill it with the best gasoline, you change the oil, and if something starts to go wrong, you take it to the garage right away. And yet, if you are thirty pounds overweight, you probably pay no attention. You say, "Well, the people in my family are big." Or perhaps you smoke and your favorite food is well-marbled steak. You think exercise is something for other people.

How can this be? How can you take better care of your car's engine than of your own health?

You know the phone number of an aunt, your social security number, your license plate number. But if I ask you, "What is your blood pressure?" you will probably answer, "I don't know. My doctor knows." "What is your cholesterol level? What about your blood sugar?" "I don't know; I never checked that."

So you rely on the physician who has a list of all the numbers that have to do with your health. But what does that change? Does it change your weight, the fat and salt and sugar you eat, or the number of cigarettes you smoke? Does it make you put on jogging shoes? You wait to consult with the doctor until a disease has gotten really severe, until you can't ignore it anymore.

BE RESPONSIBLE FOR YOUR HEART

Suppose it turns out you have diabetes. If you wait to see your doctor until the last phase of the disease, multiple organ damage—heart attack, kidney failure, even the onset of blindness or a stroke—will already have happened. Any one of these could be caused by the diabetes you didn't know you had.

You never checked yourself for diabetes. You never worried about it. You thought that what your doctor knows about you would be enough. But you don't come to see him or her often enough; you ignore warning signs until your body is severely damaged and your doctor can only patch up what's left.

I hope you can see now that going to the doctor is not enough. Trusting your doctor is not enough. Even having all the tests in the world is not enough. This is especially true if you don't know what the results are and how you must act on them. Medical tests and procedures can be useful—they have saved many lives—but they are only temporary help. The real solution lies with you, with your own awareness of and responsibility for your health.

This responsibility may involve doing some things that are difficult for you: changing your diet, stopping smoking, learning to control your inner life. But it will be worth it, I promise you. It will give you many more years of health. And you won't have to do it alone. You will have me and your own doctor to help you every step of the way.

To see how you can begin taking control of your health, read on.

GETTING THE BEST (WHILE AVOIDING THE REST) OF MODERN MEDICINE

To me, the most important aspect of medicine is not the medication itself but the patient-physician relationship. The main problem I see in modern medicine is the often unsatisfactory relationship between the patient and physician. The basic reason for this unhappy relationship is, I believe, that the physician does not know the patient as a person and vice versa. The result is a relationship that is superficial, cold—in short, professional—and not conducive to a full partnership in health.

What is the result of such a sterile relationship? To me, the worst is what can happen to the patient. Let's take a hypothetical patient, Mr. X. He comes to the doctor with a possible heart problem, say, chest pain of unknown origin. He enters his doctor's diagnostic factory, where he undergoes a series of confusing and even frightening tests. Nobody tells him what's going on, and at the end he receives the final diagnosis, which is like a label he has to wear for life. Coronary Disease, it says. So he went through the whole process from interview to diagnosis without a clear understanding of why the tests were performed, what the tests mean, what the diagnosis means, what the medical implications are, and what he can expect of the rest of his life.

The Patient-Physician Relationship

Mr. X's story typifies to me the work of modern medicine—the mechanization of what should be a very human and interactive process. After all, the patient and the physician are supposedly working together toward a common goal—the patient's health—yet all we see is separation between the two.

Even worse, because of the lack of connection between the doctor and the patient, the patient's chances to get better are reduced. The doctor is just too busy and uncomfortable with one-on-one contact to follow up, to explain. So the patient is left to wander around alone and get sick again, because only his *symptom* has been taken care of; he has not been healed.

Whose fault is all this? No one's, really. The fact is that not only are doctors too busy, but they also have not been trained to interact with patients in a way that will set the stage for true healing. This lack of human interaction and connection is costing lives every day. A recent study showed that three out of every four people at risk for developing heart disease could be identified if health-care providers had the time and resources to counsel patients routinely on proper nutrition, cholesterol, and other risk factors. It's hard to believe, but the study showed that only about half of all patients who have significant risk factors are counseled by their physicians.

The study indicates time constraint as the main reason for the lack of counseling, but I believe it goes deeper than that, back to the fact that few patients have a true relationship with their doctors. After all, how can a relationship be healthy if it is based primarily on the identification of disease?

I remember in my own medical training that we shared shower facilities and meals with other residents and hospital employees. During meals there were often discussions about all matters of life and death—except those having to do with us. Our personal feelings and internal struggles never came up. Even in those early days, professional isolation was the rule. No wonder so many doctors maintain a distance from their patients. Yet most patients know immediately when a physician attempts to hide behind a wall of emotional defenses.

I recently spoke to Marian, who was extremely fearful about some tests she would be taking the next day. She told me her cardiologist had come into the room and rapidly rattled off a list of tests, including an angiogram. "If a coronary artery is narrow, we will do an angioplasty," he told her offhandedly. "A surgeon will be on standby, because if there are any complications, you will need open-heart surgery." As Marian looked at her doctor in shock, trying to think of questions to ask, he was already out the door. "By the way," he added, "you should lose twenty pounds and stop smoking." And he took off.

In my opinion, this sort of attitude toward the patient does not serve either the patient or the physician. To me the most fundamental step toward health and healing consists of empowering the patient. In this respect, the physician assumes a spiritual role and should work to increase the patient's awareness of the healing power of nature. The idea is that the seat of spirituality within does the healing, so the physician is, in essence, evoking that spirit. This essence of spirituality is, in my view, an essential component of health. *Mens sana in corpore sano*. Health of mind and body are one.

Patient Empowerment

There are three fundamental areas in which the physician can be particularly helpful to patients.

The first area is helping the patient to face reality by clearly giving what facts are available and dissolving the screen of illusion. In my experience, honesty and openness are the quickest first aid for fear. Fear makes people exaggerate or minimize discomfort. It makes them jump into action too soon—or, conversely, paralyzes them in indecision when their lives are at stake.

I believe that patients have a right to know as much as possible about what is going on with their own health. I believe patients heal more quickly when they have this exchange of information with their doctors. The reduction of fear can allow the patient's own wisdom (including wisdom of the body) to participate in

decisions regarding healing. I have seen many people die because they were not informed.

Mrs. Boniface, one of my exceptional heart patients, told me
what she expected of a doctor at one of our first meetings. "I like
a physician who comes in and sits down and talks to me for a
while," she said. "Most doctors just mumble and bless me and
say they'll see me tomorrow. They don't sit down and ask me
how I'm doing and explain things. You know, if I'm going under
the knife, I want to sit and talk to the doctor. I want to say, 'Hey,
look, guy, you have my life in your hands. I'm at your mercy. So
I have to have trust in you.' "

A second area where the physician can be helpful to the patient is with the family. At times of great emotional stress, decisions must be made that may leave their mark for all the years
to come. As close as the physician may be to the patient, in most
cases he or she still has more emotional distance than the family.
Not only can the physician help to keep family members informed as they make their decisions, but he or she can also be a
friend and guide them emotionally, as seems appropriate, from
the store of personal experiences, and even urge them, as I often
do, to tell the patient whatever they would want him or her to
know before death. The physician can care for the emotional
well-being of the family in very specific ways when the patient
cannot.

I remember Walter, a dignified sixty-eight-year-old man who
never showed his feelings, even after cancer had invaded his
body. Walter's wife, Edna, was one of my heart patients, but
whenever I was in the hospital, I always sat with him for a while.
Each time I told him that I admired him for his strength and
courage. One day I learned from one of his physicians that Walter had gotten worse. The next day his wife had an appointment
with me. I told her that Walter was seriously ill and that I
thought she should go see him and tell him of her love. She

began to cry, then told me she was going straight to the hospital. I felt the need to call Walter's son. I explained to him that maybe I was invading personal territory, but I thought he should speak to his father. There was a pause, and then Walter's son asked me, "What should I say?"

I thought for a moment, then spoke from my heart. "Tell him how much you love him," I said, "in whatever way seems best. Also tell him that, whatever he decides to do, it is all right with you. Give him permission to be free."

Walter died a few days later. At the funeral, with tears in their eyes, his wife and son told me how grateful they were that I had made it easier for them to tell Walter what was in their hearts.

A third area in which physicians can be helpful is in honoring the patient's decisions and trusting the patient's judgments. The physician can give moral support when it is most crucial. More than once I have let my patients know, for instance, that I honor and support their choice to live or die. I want to know what *they* want and to support them physically, emotionally, and spiritually to the very best of my ability and with all my heart. The whole person brings his or her body into my office; therefore, it is the whole person with whom I am in relationship as a physician.

The Physician as Teacher

Perhaps all these areas can be summed up in what I am growing to see as the physician's most important role, that of educator, teacher of health. Who teaches patients how to be well? No one. They usually learn through disease; yet the lesson may lead to invalidism or even death. Therefore, I believe that a big part of the physician's job is to become a teacher. The patient sees the physician as powerful, so he or she has a great power over the patient. Every meeting with a patient becomes an opportunity to teach, using heart models, posters, diagrams, booklets, videotapes. I've found that my patients appreciate this information very much and that, just by having information about their illness, they become less fearful.

There are other, simpler ways doctors can begin to improve relationships with patients. For example, the patient's first contact is usually through the physician's secretary by phone. Physicians should encourage their secretaries to communicate with a friendly voice, a warm disposition, and a sincere concern. As for the doctors, when meeting a patient, they should be sure to make eye contact. Questions in the patient's mind must be answered. How much does this doctor care about me, the patient wonders. How much is he or she interested in my well-being and in helping me? That is all the patient wants to know. The initial bond is at the human level.

As for the patient, it goes without saying that the patient should take care of himself. She should respect her body and mind, try to maintain a reasonable weight, eat judiciously, keep active, and make periodic visits to the doctor for routine tests. But just as important, or perhaps more important, the patient must maintain an active role and be willing to work with the physician wholeheartedly. He should respect the doctor and have faith that the doctor will do all that is possible and available. The patient should be willing to drop her defenses and give an accurate description of her symptoms. He should be willing to share emotions and feelings and circumstances of his life that might somehow be related to the current illness.

All this is much easier for the patient if the doctor, too, upholds the ideal of the working relationship. But how can you find such a doctor?

Finding the Right Doctor

First, don't settle for a doctor who comes from the old mold. Many doctors are uncomfortable with interaction. The most common physician profile I see is the practitioner who is reserved, alone, aloof, time-conscious, worried, concerned about looking good all the time, rarely smiling, and chronically late because he is so often overbooked at the office or tied up at the hospital with emergencies.

With such doctors, professional standards and professional dignity fill up the room until the patient disappears. They forget that we physicians don't deal with disease, we deal with people who have a disease. These doctors' professionalism acts as a barrier. It protects them from something that intimidates most of us, personal contact.

The trouble with this professional barrier is that it cuts in two directions. Not only does it shield the doctor from intimidating interaction with the patient but it can also harmfully shield the patient from the openness with the physician that she needs in order to participate in her own recovery. It prevents the patient from experiencing his own fear. Thus the patient may rather stay on drugs than get off them, rather risk death than find out test results, rather rationalize symptoms than bring them into the examining room where they might be treated. Many physicians throw up their hands at such thinking, but in general they do not acknowledge that they themselves are party to the alienation that produces such denial and delay.

Another consequence of this alienation is that many patients feel they are not seen as individuals who need help with their health but as a potential market for the medical factory's product. As a result, the patient is not in any way helped to take responsibility for his or her own health.

Assessing the Patient-Physician Relationship

How, then, can a patient choose a doctor with whom she will be able to develop a quality relationship? How can he evaluate the quality of his relationship with his present physician?

There is no surefire answer, but a good place to begin is to ask yourself the following questions (inspired by John Henry Pfifferling, founder of the Society for Professional Well-being):

• Does the doctor's office have a warm, comfortable atmosphere? Is the secretary helpful and friendly?
• Do I have the chance to comfortably express all that I feel?
• Does the doctor really listen to me?
• After communicating with my doctor, do I feel relieved or frustrated?
• Do I share with my doctor the responsibility for my own well-being?
• Am I given freedom of choice among different treatment plans?
• When in doubt, do I feel comfortable voicing my need for a second opinion?
• Does the doctor share his or her knowledge without intimidation?
• Do I feel comfortable following my doctor's advice and instructions?
• Do I perceive that my doctor is doing everything possible to help me?
• Does the relationship with my doctor fulfill my expectations and needs?

If you can answer yes to most of these questions, and if you feel comfortable with your doctor as a human being, then the two of you are ready to begin a working partnership. If you cannot answer most of these questions positively, or if for some reason you and the doctor just don't hit it off, then you should look around until you find someone you are more compatible with.

Your Responsibility as a Patient

Once you have found a doctor that you like and trust, your responsibility has not ended. In fact, in a way it has just begun, because you and the physician will be working as a team to ensure your wellness. Your responsibility starts the minute you come in the physician's office door. You must be open with your doctor, forthright; don't hold out.

You must look after your own best interest by asking questions, asking questions, asking questions. Don't worry about making your doctor blow her stack or being told he's too busy to explain everything.

You are also responsible for getting a second opinion. You are responsible for getting your own needs met by this physician—or for finding another physician who *can* meet your needs.

You are responsible for getting well, for doing everything within your power to regain your health. That may seem obvious. But you would be surprised how many patients not only wait until they are very sick before seeing a doctor but also refuse to do what they're advised. They don't take their medicine, refuse to change their lifestyles, and fail to follow their physicians' instructions.

The bottom line is that you assume responsibility for *full* participation in your own healing: It's your need; it's your work.

Open-Heart Medicine

To me, the real point of medicine is focusing on what is positive, how to make life happier and longer, and not necessarily on how to escape death, which is an unavoidable reality for us all.

I believe that it is going to become more and more easy for patients to find doctors who are willing to relate to them as people. In part this is because of the increased interest in holistic medicine, the consideration of the patient as a whole person. This entails the active participation of the patient in the learning process and the help of a team of professionals who work together to increase the patient's knowledge.

Thus, a dietitian would provide the patient with basic information about food and proper nutrition. An exercise physiologist would teach the patient the benefit of cautious exercise. A psychologist would instruct the patient about meditation and relaxation exercises. He or she may also lead cardiac support group discussion sessions. Although such a team approach to health is not yet common, it is becoming more so. Speak to your doctor about the possibilities of enlisting such a team in your recovery process.

By learning about the mind-body relationship, by practicing meditation/relaxation techniques, you can discover the self-healing mechanisms within yourself. Such empowerment does not imply any disregard of modern medical techniques, especially diagnostic techniques; rather it raises your level of understanding and thus promotes your ability to take better care of yourself in partnership with your physician.

The truth is that most heart patients feel powerless. To be an exceptional heart patient, you must be power*ful*, you must take full charge. If this seems sometimes as if you are taking some of the responsibility from your doctor, so be it. One doctor said that the man who is his own physician has a fool for a doctor. Writer Tom Ferguson rephrased that maxim: The person who does not act as his own physician, who does not take responsibility for his case, who does not keep a close eye on all phases of his body and his treatment, who does not ask good questions, who does not exercise a high degree of choice and control, is the biggest fool of all.

SEVEN KEYS TO A HEALTHY HEART

Why wait for a heart attack to happen? Wouldn't it be fantastic to prevent it and lead a healthy, normal life, treasuring the miracle of health? The truth is that whatever your heart's level of healthiness or illness, even in the case of advanced heart disease, there's a great deal you can do to keep your heart healthy or heal it.

The most important step you can take is to make a commitment to practice daily the seven keys to a healthy heart:

1. Respect your body. This precept is fundamental. Maintain the weight you had when you were eighteen years old (if you were healthy then). Follow the proper diet; be active. Learn to live without crutches: cigarettes, alcohol, and drugs.

2. Take time to relax every day. Relaxation is not a luxury; it is a need. You may relax reading, listening to music, painting, gardening.

3. Accept, respect, and appreciate yourself. This key is fundamental to a healthy heart. Accept yourself, respect yourself, and appreciate yourself as a whole, including those parts of you that other people may have said are not okay.

4. Share your deepest feelings. Be honest with yourself and others. Share your true self. This is the greatest gift you can give to another person.

5. Establish life goals. Choose goals in harmony with your work and personal values and focus on them, investing your life with meaning. The achievement of the goal is not as important as the process.

6. Love yourself and others unconditionally. Love is the greatest healing power in the universe. The pathway to love is forgiveness.

7. Nourish your spiritual self. Become aware of the fact that you are not only a body but also a spirit.

These keys will be examined in more detail in future chapters.

Chapter Three

YOUR MIND

AND YOUR HEART

The brain is capable of holding a conversation
with the body that ends in death.
—Russian proverb

*T*hey were a very happy couple, devoted to each other. Two years after their fiftieth anniversary, the wife developed cancer of the breast and died. Two or three months afterward, her husband had a heart attack and also died.

What is the explanation for this double, and not uncommon, tragedy? There is no way to know for certain, but all too often I see a very close relationship between a stressful event and illness. A recent patient of mine, Bernice, who had raised 120 foster children, was referred to me by the surgeon who had performed coronary bypass on her after a seemingly sudden heart attack. I thought I had gotten all the information pertinent to her heart attack from her surgeon, but I found out something more when we met in the conference room in my office. It seemed that Bernice had been given a child by a social worker, raised the child for eight years, and then had to give the child up. She had done so much for him already that it was like giving up her own son. But the rules were inflexible, and she obeyed them. Six weeks later she had a heart attack.

A coincidence? Maybe. But the short time between these events is curious indeed. It is becoming increasingly well known that the mind and the body work together. The mind can affect the heart to the point of creating heart disease.

But this news is not all negative. Quite the contrary. Just as the mind can create disease, under the right circumstances it can cure disease.

I'll never forget Van, a patient of mine who had open-heart surgery twice. After the second operation he developed lung cancer, for which he received radiation therapy and the verdict that he only had six months to live. I told him that no physician can give verdicts and urged him to refuse this one. I then advised him to read a book on visualization techniques for cancer patients. He did so and confessed to me that during radiation treatments he visualized the therapy as a powerful tool to kill all the cancer cells in his body. He urged the invisible rays on, saying to himself, "Kill that sucker!"

To the surprise of his oncologist, but not to himself or to me, Van is still cancer-free after three years. There is no evidence of a tumor; only scar tissue remains.

Another exceptional patient I remember is Elaine, who at the age of five had her leg amputated. At the age of twenty she developed lung cancer and after surgery underwent radiation that damaged her heart. Thus, she had to go through yet another operation, a heart transplant.

As I spoke to Elaine for the first time on the phone, I visualized her sitting in a wheelchair in a nursing home, eking out her pain-ridden days. But when she first came in to visit me I realized how wrong my assumptions had been. I saw before me a vibrant twenty-four-year-old woman, with the face and voice of a happy, mature, spiritually fulfilled person. She is happily married, has a child, and works full-time. I can honestly say that Elaine is one of the happiest people I have ever met.

Then there is Steven, a man in his forties who developed cardiomyopathy (a wasting of the heart muscle) and was told he would die soon. To compound the tragedy, Steven was married and had children. His physician finally said there was nothing more to be done but undergo a heart transplant. My friend accepted that as the only answer to extending his life. While recovering from the operation, Steven learned that his wife wanted to divorce him. Now even his family, the most intimate treasure of his life, was destroyed.

But Steven didn't give up. Somehow, he found the strength to recover, and after some time he happily remarried. He also trained his body, became far healthier and stronger than he had been before his illness, and went on to win several gold medals in the Olympics reserved for cardiac transplant patients. He had become a spiritual giant.

How can we account for these remarkable recoveries? The skill of the surgeons, certainly. But there is something more: A strength of will enabled these exceptional patients to use their minds to help heal their bodies. Although this mind-body connection is becoming better known, it is true that many, if not most, physicians still view the mind and the body as separate, and distinct, entities.

HOW YOUR DOCTOR
VIEWS HEART DISEASE

We physicians, cardiologists in particular, have spent most of our time training to recognize and identify disease. In fact, I don't recall ever having been trained in the United States or in Europe in anything other than diagnosis of disease. As a practicing physician I was inevitably confronted with the fact that some people recover and others don't. But I also observed that some of the people who recover are not supposed to recover according to our predictions. I began to ask myself whether there were values at play beyond the ones traditional medicine identifies as key to the development or reduction of heart disease.

According to physicians in cardiology literature, the facts are relatively simple. There are a number of basic conditions that predispose one toward hardening of the arteries, which is the major element responsible for heart attack. These include high blood pressure, high cholesterol, cigarette smoking, lack of exercise, diabetes, obesity, and stress. Other contributing factors include being born male, increasing age, and a family history of heart disease. These are the fundamentals. They are so fundamental, in fact, that they are known as the heart disease risk factors.

Stress and the Heart

Calling these risk factors means that if you stay away from cigarette smoking, if your blood pressure is controlled, if your weight is regular and you are physically fit, then the risk of heart disease and heart attack is significantly reduced.

Statistically, all this is true, but people are not statistics. It has been my experience that emotional stress is very important in determining the risk of coronary artery disease and thus heart attacks.

Let's say we have a smoker who is at risk for heart disease, or let's say he's already had a heart attack. What do we do? We take his cigarettes away and tell him not to smoke. But we're just removing an effect, aren't we? The cause, why the person uses tobacco in the first place, is not dealt with at all. Why is this person smoking?

Or let's say a person is overweight and we tell her to lose thirty or forty pounds. But why is she overweight? Why is she eating so much? Likewise, if someone has high blood pressure, we know how to treat it, but, in over 90 percent of the cases, we don't know the cause. Oh, we do know from experiments that one of the basic factors responsible for raising blood pressure is peripheral vasoconstriction. This means that the smaller blood vessels, the arterioles, have squeezed themselves down, causing unusual resistance to the flow of blood and thus raising blood pressure. But why is this constriction happening? What is causing the arterioles to squeeze themselves shut?

To me these are very important questions. To me it seems obvious that we doctors should not limit ourselves to treating the effects of disease. We can't eliminate these effects anyway, most of the time, without eliminating the primary reason for the events. To talk about real treatment, real cure, we have to talk about the whole person. When you bring a sickness in your body to me, you are bringing the last and most recent evidence of something gone wrong. And you are telling me, my friend, that you have already been paying a price for quite a while. Your symptoms are the bill; your high blood pressure, angina, diabetes, heart attack, they are what you've bought.

What you've been spending in the meantime is the health and well-being of your mind and feelings. You may come in physically fit from jogging but emotionally unfit: mad, scared, holding a grudge, depressed, despairing. This is costing you in two ways. First, you have to live all the time in that bad emotional weather. Second, left alone, that kind of unfitness will cause disease.

Who Gets Sick?

I'll have more to say about ways to get out of that bad weather later on in the book. For now I want to get back to the risk factors. Some of the risk factors for heart attack you can't do anything about, such as being born male, getting older, or having a family history of heart disease. Others you can completely change. You can give up smoking, lose weight, and so on. In further chapters I'll show you ways that exceptional heart patients have managed to change their risk factors and increase their own wellness.

But risk factors are only a part of the story. The truth is that only 50 percent of people who have heart problems have even some of the risk factors. What about the people who don't have these risk factors? What is it that they think or do that makes them cardiac patients? What is it in the way they live that can alter the anatomy of their hearts? And even those who have all the risk factors may have larger problems that go beyond easy clinical definitions.

I believe all the risk factors can be traced to deeper lifestyle problems. Lifestyle and attitude are the source of the problem, not the smoking or high blood pressure or cholesterol. In my view, everything begins in the mind.

In modern medicine, unfortunately, all we look at are the statistics. We are oriented toward emphasizing what is bad for your heart instead of pointing to what is good for it. The risk factors are all negative. What about the positive factors? What about the elements that make it *less* likely that you will develop heart disease? For me these are very important. They include joy, happiness, peace of mind, serenity, love, self-love, and the ability to share yourself with others.

A MIND-BODY MODEL OF HEART DISEASE

Recently a patient was referred to my office by another cardiologist. Eugene was vibrantly healthy-looking, lean, fit. I learned that two years earlier this fifty-three-year-old man had been found to have a critical narrowing of the two major branches of the left coronary artery. He had been advised to have surgery but refused. Instead, he followed Dr. Dean Ornish's 10 percent fat diet, lost seventy-five pounds, and after that came to my office. He told me that his original cardiologist told him that his thallium stress test, approximately a year after he started his program, was normal. The cardiologist was very perplexed.

I could understand why when I saw Eugene's original coronary angiogram. Judging from the types of lesions I saw, this patient needed surgery, and I was extremely surprised to see him coming into my office alive, much less smiling and without symptoms.

So the question is, how did Eugene's heart heal itself? I believe that there must be a healing mechanism within not just the heart but the whole body. Moreover, I believe that some people have a pattern of disease that they hold in their minds. I remember a patient who had a narrowing of the right coronary artery that was shaped like a triangle. I did an angioplasty, but unfortunately the lesion came back two months later. I advised a second angioplasty, but the patient refused, opting instead for surgery. Two months after the bypass surgery, his chest pain recurred, and the angiogram showed, in the bypass itself, exactly the same triangle-shaped lesion that had occurred twice in the original artery. I was left without a clear explanation as to how this happened, but it was evident that this patient's body knew how to create the narrowing of an artery.

The Mind as a Healer

But just as our minds may know how to create disease, they have the capacity to heal. The body, in a sense, has a mind of its own. When you think about it, this shouldn't seem so strange. After all, hypnosis has shown that the body is obedient to the commands it receives from the mind. It can raise a blister on skin that no flame ever touched; it can cause a person to shake and chatter with cold when the room temperature is comfortably warm.

The connection between the mind and body is something we've always been aware of, yet we have felt it needed to be proved by science before we could act on it or talk about it. All doctors have had miraculous cures, and, though they make us feel good personally, they are scientifically embarrassing to the medical community.

My own experience with the mind-body relationship has caused me to change my ways of dealing with many patients. For instance, I am much more solicitous of comatose patients, because I now know that they understand me when I speak to them, even though they are unconscious. I tell such patients how much I care about them, how much I love them and want to help them. I tell them that if they would like to get better they can, that it is their choice.

David was an eighteen-year-old student who experienced a skull fracture and went into a coma following a motorcycle accident. Seeing David apparently lifeless on a respirator, partially disfigured, was discouraging. His father and other family members were often at bedside. I always recommended that they talk to David, touch him and kiss him as if he were alert. As for myself, in my daily rounds I told him repeatedly, "David, you can make it!"

A month later David regained consciousness. Then, with rehabilitation, he went on to almost full recovery. Four years later he came to my office with his wife and child.

I am also more careful when dealing with very ill patients, and much more respectful of the fact that their wellness is their own choice. I have come to believe something that may shock you. I think things sometimes go wrong with patients because they want them to.

I remember Hilary, whom I brought back after a massive heart attack. He begged me, "Doctor, I want to die. Please let me die!"

But his family was not ready yet. Hilary stopped eating. I continued the IV fluids, but his decision was irrevocable. So, like a melting candle, he wasted until a few days later his wife and children, seeing that he was already taking action, told him it was all right to go. He died peacefully.

On the other side there was tall, slender, gray-haired Carol, who always held herself regally and spoke softly, her blue eyes looking out from an oval face that developed a slight tremor when she spoke. Though she seemed aloof, her smile was always warm and beautiful. Until one day . . .

"Stroke," I noted in my journal. "One leg is becoming gangrenous. Her lungs are congested, and, in my opinion, she is giving up."

In fact, when Carol's daughter talked to me shortly after the stroke, I told her that her mother was seriously ill and that, worst of all, she was giving up. I thought a minute and then added, "She is probably waiting for your permission to go, and she is giving you time to accept her decision." The daughter started crying. I hugged her and said, "I don't want to hurt you, but in my opinion, that's the truth. Of course, we will continue to do everything possible to enable her to go home, but I don't see any will to live in her eyes."

Carol had an amputation; the remaining stump above the knee was blue and cold. But her eye contact gave me a little handle, a handle of love, with which I could pull her along. Every day her eyes would follow me like a camera when I was in her room. Because she had one tube in her mouth and another in her nose, the most she could manage as a greeting was a small smile from one corner of her mouth, but I saw it!

"What do you have in mind?" I asked her one day. "I want to know what you want."

That day she was evasive and would not look at me. I thought she was confirming a decision to die. But the next day she fooled me. "I want to go home," she told me. And she did. This amazing woman, who was wearing out a team of nurses per shift in the hospital, now is managing like a dream at home with the equivalent of a half-time nurse. Carol, I realized, had needed some time to make up her mind whether or not she wanted to die.

Thinking Makes It So

What greater proof do we need that the individual mind and body are not only linked but in constant communication with each other than these histories of patients who take the option of death or, in the face of death, life? A sickness may be a patient's desire to become ill, and finally, if his life has no meaning, to leave life altogether. Who are we to judge? Sometimes life hands us a problem which we would rather die than experience, so we do.

More and more it becomes evident that, with many illnesses, thinking makes it so, and thus we doctors must be very, very careful how we influence what our patients think. In fact, I believe that some patients don't know how sick they are until their doctors tell them. I remember a patient who came to my office seemingly in perfect health. She had a minor discomfort in her belly, so I did an ultrasound exam. Unfortunately, the diagnosis was possible cancer of the gallbladder. This patient was hospitalized and, after an extensive workup, her medical team reached the same conclusion. Naturally, she had to undergo treatment, and within two months she died. I am sure that if I had not found her gallbladder problem, she would have lived much longer.

Likewise, I believe it is possible that some people with a heart problem overreact to the diagnosis and die of it, while others who have the same disease take the necessary steps to overcome it. The truth is that if we can change our interpretation of an event, we can change how we perceive reality itself.

Naturally, I am not saying that you shouldn't go to the doctor for minor discomforts. What I am saying is that when the diagnosis is frightening panic can take over. It can become more difficult to find a way to heal ourselves. This is why I am opposed to stark predictions, such as "You have six months to live" or "You will never walk again." To my way of thinking, if a patient is able to maintain his or her independence in thinking, and still sees the disease as curable, that will increase longevity and the chances of recovery. In a word, do not succumb to the verdict of your physician. Allow your vision of yourself to remain pure.

This can work the other way as well. I remember a patient who had an enlarged heart and was getting progressively weaker, losing the ability to do even the most normal things. With some hesitance, I advised him to start cardiac rehabilitation. Well, that advice had a profound impact. Before, he had believed he was too sick, but just the idea that he could rehabilitate himself gave him enough strength to go to the gym two or three times a week. Whereas he had been frequently confined to bed, now he was active. There was a new light in his eyes. His heart got stronger. He became able to walk and to exercise longer.

What changed? The only thing that changed, in my view, was his belief that he could improve himself. He discovered that he was not at the end of the line, that other tools were available, and he willingly took those tools to heart.

The Body Knows How to Heal

I wonder how many tools there are that we never use in our lives. How many times do we not tune into the possibilities for wellness that are beyond the level of our awareness? I believe that the body has an innate, divine intelligence that is capable of self-healing without medical intervention. When you have a cut finger, the blood stops flowing. Who or what stopped the bleeding? Not your doctor, not any medication. A few weeks later when you look at your finger, the cut is gone. There is no scar; it's completely healed. Your body has healed itself.

Modern science is just beginning to understand the natural mechanisms that underlie any sort of healing, from a cut finger to cancer and heart disease. This link between the mind and the body is now evident in the field of psychoneuroimmunology. This mouthful of a word is the science that explores the connection between the mind, the nervous system, and the immune system. In this view, the mind and body are not only connected but inseparable. Research has shown that the brain produces special molecules, called neuropeptides, which interact with every cell of the body, including those of the immune system. Every emotion produces these substances, and every cell of the body is receptive to them. The emotions, in a very real sense, are not just in the mind but in the body as well.

Every day exciting discoveries are being made in this field. Joan Borysenko, author of *Guilt Is the Teacher, Love Is the Lesson*, tells of an experiment in which researchers trained mice to shut down their own immune systems when given apple juice. A study at the University of Pennsylvania that evaluated Harvard graduates found that the more pessimistic the Harvard men were, the more likely they were to develop disease.

Although the physical mechanisms behind many of these startling findings have yet to be discovered, there is some evidence that mood can affect the activity of crucial cells in the immune system. Thus, as Deepak Chopra believes, when we are happy we are actually physiologically different than when we are depressed.

But no matter what future research shows, it is clear that, however they work, these links between the body and the mind can make all the difference between health and sickness. Health lies in a balanced immune system. The equilibrium may be re-established or maintained by behavioral techniques, such as meditation, visualization, or relaxation. This is an example of the power of behavior on the immune system. Isn't it a fantastic power to become aware of?

RETHINKING YOUR NEGATIVE BELIEFS ABOUT HEART DISEASE

Although they may not be aware of it, the exceptional heart patients I've interviewed have made use of this innate power. They know that labels influence judgment and refuse to be la-beled as cardiac patients. A patient who categorizes himself as such places himself in a class of people who are incapacitated, deprived of autonomy, invalids. Yet on many occasions this is not the reality. If patients accept the category in which they are placed, they become disempowered.

Conversely, the conception that a heart attack is an experi-ence that we can overcome favors a more positive outcome.

The truth is that cardiac patients who think of themselves as invalids still have reservoirs of energy in their hearts and bodies that are never used because they don't perceive them. They never bother to look for them. A cardiac patient refraining from sports because she's been told and believes the heart can't take such activity may worsen her condition with the very inactivity she may think is helping.

Such learned helplessness is implied by strictures preventing cardiac patients from mowing the lawn, shoveling snow, playing tennis, and making love. The categories of "supposed to" and "not supposed to" are, like all distinctions, artificial.

Unfortunately, society often buys into this negativity. Patients of mine who underwent bypass surgery have been refused employment because their bosses viewed them as potential liabilities. But, as I pointed out in one such case, a heart patient is a more reliable employee than many other people. After all, he must take good care of himself, minding his diet, exercise, and stress levels.

The results of negative belief may be even greater. For example, nearly 6 percent of all heart attacks, and probably 24 percent of heart attacks in those below the age of thirty-five, occur in people whose angiograms show normal coronary arteries. Yet if the artery goes into prolonged spasm, the effect may be a heart attack, and it is just as deadly or incapacitating as if it were caused by a clot. Likewise, the most common cause of death in people who have a heart attack is an irregular heartbeat known as ventricular fibrillation. This arrhythmia may also be caused by an electrical imbalance, which can be linked to emotional stress.

Even intense fear, then, may cause cardiac arrest or ventricular fibrillation. In other words, we can become so frightened that our hearts will find it easier to stop than to continue beating.

I honestly believe that heart disease is essentially a disease of self, caused by self, and is made worse by the belief that we are its victims. If I had to summarize the negative and incorrect beliefs held by many people about heart disease, that would be at the top of the list.

Another misconception holds that the possibilities for recovery are limited. There are people who have become athletic champions after a heart problem. There are lives that have been reformed completely after a heart attack. If you are willing to learn from the experience, understand why you went through it, find the causative factors, and correct them, then the experience you thought was negative will become a path to recovery, self-improvement, and growth.

Sometimes a heart attack can bring the family together,

awakening the need for love and support that was dormant in the past. Or the person who used to be shy, isolated, and lonely suddenly opens his heart to others, revealing his own humanity and innocence. He heals his own heart. The experience of the heart attack then becomes an opportunity to improve one's life.

Chapter Four

"BUT IT CAN'T
HAPPEN TO ME!"

There is nothing the body suffers that the soul may not profit by.
—George Meredith

t has been my experience that we often change when a disease affects us. I've seen patients who've had heart attacks undergo radical transformations, and I can't help wondering why. I've seen them do the expected things, such as lose weight, stop smoking, and begin regular exercise. But I've also seen them change from within. In essence, after the heart attack they look at life differently. They have had the opportunity to face death and return as victors.

After the initial shock and pain of the heart attack, such patients regain an inner strength. They rediscover life; they find the joy of smelling flowers, looking at the blue sky, taking a walk, breathing the fresh air, listening to the wind. They notice new flowers blooming, and spring returns to their hearts.

They lose the feeling of being scattered and regain the ability to be centered. Their attention moves from the outer life to the life within. They focus on that part of themselves that never dies, the spiritual part, and develop a sense of connectedness to that spirit.

FROM VICTIM TO VICTOR

The lesson they learned from their heart attacks has shaken these patients to the core. Now they must find an answer to compelling questions such as, What is the meaning of my life? Why am I here? What does God want from me? How can I contribute? What can I become?

As I look into the eyes of each of these patients, I see the serenity of a person who has discovered a new truth and believes it wholeheartedly. She has learned to listen to the small inner voice that will guide her from now on through a life invested with meaning, to a new beginning.

I believe that one reason a heart attack can so profoundly change someone is that, more than any other illness, it launches a direct assault on our concept of who we are. The truth is that a heart attack is not just a physical event but an emotional and spiritual one too. The heart attack sets in progress profound changes that affect every cell in the body. There are hormonal changes, physical and psychological changes, emotional and spiritual changes, that all take place when a person is suddenly taken from a state of seeming well-being to the edge of life.

Adding to the stress is the fact that the full reality of what has occurred often does not set in until the heart attack is well in progress. Here's how Martin, a fifty-year-old dentist, described it: "It was very simple. I was sitting in my office, treating a patient. I suddenly started sweating and feeling very weak. I finished interviewing the patient and sent him home. I called my doctor and told him I was having a coronary and I'd be right over. I made a bank deposit and closed my office. Then I got in the cab, told the driver, 'Take me to Grand Hospital.' I got to the hospital and went right upstairs to the cardiac unit. The doctor started to do an ECG, then he took a look at me and said, 'Let's get him into the ICU.' They tried to find a vein to start an IV, but they couldn't find one and I collapsed."

Martin was lucky. Despite his delays, he made it to the hospital on time; many victims of heart attack don't. In fact, I'd say that the greatest danger for a patient who is experiencing a heart attack is the delay from the beginning of symptoms to the arrival at the hospital. Believe it or not, the average time is between 2.9 and 5.1 hours, which explains why 50 to 80 percent of deaths occur within four hours of symptoms. The reason for delay may be denial, or fear, or anxiety: "This can't be happening to me!" Or perhaps it is rationalization: "It's just indigestion" or "This can't be a heart attack, I'm too young!"

Yet every minute of delay can be crucial. Provided that the victim gets to the hospital on time, medical personnel can apply thrombolytic agents, substances that dissolve the blood clot, literally stopping the heart attack in progress.

The Wounded Heart

Once you have reached the hospital, everything in your life changes. Suddenly you are confined to a hospital bed, immobilized by IVs, needles, machines, and monitoring systems. You are told when you can and can't leave the bed, even to go to the washroom, and what and what not to eat. It is a shocking and frightening experience. "It was disorienting," said William, a hard-driving businessman who developed a heart attack after repeated episodes of chest pain. "It's strange when you're healthy as a horse one day, and then, out of the blue, you get leveled like this. You become helpless and dependent on other people. You learn that no man is an island. You always need other people."

But gradually, like William, you will adjust to your new reality. At least a great number of people do. You realize, once you have been disconnected from the machines and all the monitoring systems, that you are standing up by yourself, you are breathing by yourself, you have normal blood pressure and heartbeat all by yourself. You begin to regain the independence that we all crave in life.

After the initial flush of autonomy comes another period, what I think of as the wounded heart phase. You have the memory of what happened in the past and a fear of the future. What really happened? you wonder. How bad is my heart? Will I be able to work again? Will I live to see my children grow up? These questions can be overwhelming at times. Even when there is no rational basis for these fears, they occur, and they are perfectly normal. "I'm always afraid," one patient told me after her heart attack. "I have this fear in my mind that I'm going to die. That I'm not going to wake up in the morning. This is the way I feel all the time, ever since my heart attack." Another patient spoke of hoping that "somehow I was going to find out that this was just kind of a cruel joke. That it was not permanent and that I would get over it soon."

Return to Life

After the patient has completely stabilized, we perform an angiogram to discover the extent of blockage. For some patients minimal disease is revealed, so treatment by medication will be sufficient. For others there is localized narrowing in the major branch of a coronary artery, and a balloon angioplasty will usually control the problem. But for others the disease is diffuse, and bypass surgery will be necessary.

Following this phase of the heart attack, and recovery from surgery if it was performed, there is what I call a return to life.

You come back home to your family, to your dear ones. There, maybe for the first time in your life, you sense how much love surrounds you, how much your spouse and children missed you, how much your friends care. You receive so many hugs that tears come to your eyes, tears of joy because the storm is over. Many emotional barriers that surrounded you are now broken. You are glad beyond words to be back and ready to begin your new life.

You will still have worries; you would not be normal if you didn't. In my experience the primary worry is about dying. Because you've been confronted by a heart attack, you are overwhelmed by the idea that another one may be lethal. Or you want to know, How long will my life be? What will happen to my job? What role will I have in my family? I used to be the center of the family, the provider, and now I don't know if I will be able to fulfill that promise. Any heart problem thus becomes a highly charged issue that is a magnet for fear.

In some cases this phase leads to depression. Frank was shocked after his surgery to find that his wife was leaving him. ''I became so severely depressed I wanted to sleep the whole day,'' he related later. ''In my mind I became Cecil B. De Mille. I manufactured and produced the most incredible film in my mind, a film based on every failure of my past and projection of the hopelessness of my future. I did the most incredible job of undoing myself. Finally, I went to a psychiatric hospital for three weeks.''

There are also questions that relate to the feeling of your own integrity. When you look in the mirror, each time you take a shower, you will see this scar running the length of your chest. This can cause the unpleasant memories to surface. Especially for women the scar can trigger fears of loss of attractiveness and femininity. I've known some patients who, even with the most supportive husbands, feared abandonment when they looked at their scars. In addition to the psychological problems, there is also, sometimes, pain at the site of the incision, or itching.

Some patients feel guilt. They blame themselves for not having eaten properly, not having exercised, having had an unhealthy lifestyle, and they look on their heart troubles as their fault. Others may tend to blame other people, or circumstances: "My boss was pushing too hard"; "I worked too many hours." I feel it is unproductive to blame either yourself or others; rather it is necessary to take responsibility for what has happened to you and, even more important, what *will* happen.

At this time many patients begin to restrict their lives out of fear. They become afraid to exercise as they used to, or to make love, or to live in any way as they did before the heart attack. The way out of these worries is to join a rehabilitation program, learning to live actively again under supervision. Above all it is important to avoid physical and emotional invalidism.

How to Recover

How you think of yourself at this point becomes critical. Do you look at yourself as a broken vase which has been patched, with loss of integrity and unity, to be coddled and carefully watched over so it won't crack again? Or do you see yourself as someone whose heart is now strong, having recovered completely? Someone who is far richer now because you have learned from this experience how precious life is, how vulnerable all humans are, and how important it is to believe in your own values? In the first case the disease becomes a reason for giving up. In the second the disease is a step toward personal growth. In the first case the illness has destroyed a life. In the second it has fortified it.

James, a forty-nine-year-old exceptional heart patient, went through most of the emotional changes I have just described. "I was distressed," he told me, "overwhelmed. I felt like someone had punched me in the gut, and I stayed that way for sixty to ninety days. Then I started thinking I didn't want to live that way. So I found out about the Zipper Club, a support group for people who had bypass surgery. Talking to those people really helped. Then I started going to conferences that talked about alternative lifestyles and that sort of thing. I think there's more than one way to do any different thing."

The Vulnerable Period

It is during this vulnerable period that the physician can help the patient look at his or her heart in a way that is encouraging. I think it's important to tell the patient something like this: "You had a heart attack, but your heart is recovering, you are strong, there is a lot of energy left in you, and you can have a meaningful life." These are vital words, particularly when the patient is feeling loss of control. The physician and patient working in partnership can achieve major progress at this stage.

I believe that, after a heart attack or a bypass operation, our priorities change. One man I read about described this change quite honestly: "I've lost my desire to become president of another company, but I miss the challenge." I've noticed that many of my own patients are very eager to resume work, and I always encourage that aspect of life for self-image and general well-being.

From the beginning of the disease, I put myself in my patients' place. I imagine how great must be their joy when they wake up from surgery. I've greeted patients after surgery on many occasions. They are still intubated and can't talk, but our eyes meet, and I express all my love to them, showing my happiness for their courage. So it is a silent conversation when they look at me, often with a smile in their eyes because I was the one who found their heart problem.

I hope that everything in this book will help you to avoid becoming a heart patient, or, if you have or develop heart disease, that you will refuse to become a cardiac cripple and instead allow the illness to become an opportunity for growth. Despite all the negative aspects, I do believe that a heart attack or heart surgery can be growth-promoting and empowering. Look at it this way. Say you've had a heart attack. Before that happened you were completely taken up by worries, by work, financial issues, family life, and problems with intimacy. All these things prevented you from seeing your life clearly. So in the recovery phase it becomes natural to go over your life, which—unconsciously, of course—you are already addressing with Why me? questions.

I believe that the most important issue at this point is for you to become aware of the possibility of and necessity for change in your life. As you gain an understanding of the effect this illness has had on you, you should also begin to think about your resistance to change. What is preventing you from changing? I have to admit that several times I have seen patients who have had a heart attack and open-heart surgery refuse to stop smoking. What makes them resist this simple change? I remember a patient in his mid-forties who first had a heart attack, then got blockage in the arteries of both legs. Now he is able to walk less than a block, despite having had surgery in the legs twice. Would you believe that he is still smoking?

On the other side, of course, are those patients who have grown and changed as a result of their disease. I remember Mr. Adams, who after open-heart surgery seemed to be going downhill, as if he had given up. I told him that I had a lot of faith in him and that I wanted him to restart a rehabilitation program he had dropped out of in discouragement. Well, he did restart the program, and this time he stuck with it. He now looks much improved and can even work with no obvious problems. By encouraging him to go back to rehabilitation, I showed him I had faith in his recovery. This allowed him to embrace hope, which was all he needed for his body's natural healing mechanisms to take over. The other day Mr. Adams looked me in the eye and said, "Doc, make sure you don't give up on me, and I promise that I will never give up on you."

HEARTSKILL 2: SELF-CHANGE EXERCISE

The following exercise, adapted from the book *Healing with Love*, by Leonard Laskow, can be very powerful if you already have heart disease or have suffered a heart attack. It consists of several questions that can help you assess your attitude toward illness as well as your needs for change and ability to change. Even if you are still healthy, it can be useful to read over the questions.

1. What do I want to do differently?

There is no right or wrong answer to any of these questions. Maybe your answer will be "I don't want to have another heart attack." Or "I want to leave the hospital as soon as I can. I want to live a happier life, a longer life, I want to enjoy what remains of my life 100 percent."

Just answering that question puts you on the road to self-discovery and recovery. Next you might look at the reasons for this desire. There may be outer reasons, such as "I want to look better," or more important inner reasons: "I want to see my children get married"; "I want to give meaning to my life."

2. How have I contributed to the present circumstances?

You should be very gentle with yourself as you do this exercise, but honest all the same. For instance, you may recognize that smoking, improper diet, and lack of exercise have all contributed to your heart attack. Staying away from your physician for ten years, ignoring or misinterpreting the early warning signs—all of these are important issues to be addressed. But again, don't cast blame on yourself. Simply recognize your degree of responsibility in the matter. Bear in mind that even we physicians don't always know why a person had a heart attack.

The value of this exercise is that, as you see how you have contributed to the problem, you also will begin to discover that you can find your own remedies, which is a very empowering attitude, and far different from cowering on an examination table while a physician points a judgmental finger at you.

3. In what ways is this illness or situation preventing me from leading the life I want to be leading, doing the things I want to be doing? At the same time, what does it allow me to do, be, or have?

The answers to these questions are crucial because they determine whether you will perceive yourself as a victim, a cardiac cripple, or instead as someone who can become whole and healthy again. So, for instance, you may recognize that having had a heart attack prevents you from doing weight lifting or sports activities in which you have to use your muscles in a strenuous way. It may also require you to quit smoking, to stop eating fatty foods, and other seemingly difficult adjustments, but the important point is that you recognize that these are changes that you can make on your own, and that will allow you to lead the sort of life you dream about. On the other hand, you must be able to see what remains to you, the worlds of goodness that are still available. For example, you can still be a parent, and a loving and sexually active spouse; you can still grow and contribute to others. You can still accept the responsibility for your own future. Remember always that only your body has been wounded, not your spirit. If you are able to take refuge in the spiritual realm, you can find there all the strength necessary to pursue the physical and emotional changes you need.

4. Where do I want to go from here? What results do I want to create?

These questions bring you to the future as far as we can see it. For example, you may decide to start cardiac rehabilitation, to follow a stricter diet, to exercise and avoid the known risk factors. You may, in fact, decide to change your entire lifestyle, to begin doing the things you always wanted to but avoided out of fear, anxiety, or the pressures of conformity.

As you ask yourself these questions, you may find that there are many choices available to you that you never recognized before. This in turn can help you visualize the path that you want for the future. This self-examination can give you a picture of how you are now and how you really want to be.

Chapter Five

THE HEALING

PERSONALITY

Words which come from the heart enter the heart.
—Moses Ibn Ezra

*S*elf-healing can be activated by an increased sense of bodily or psychological control, achieved through biofeedback, relaxation techniques, even prayer and meditation. At the University of Iowa, for example, psychologists have prevented the increase in blood pressure that may follow coronary bypass by teaching patients exercises to reduce pain and speed recovery. At Stanford University, arthritis patients who learned relaxation techniques had a significant reduction in pain when compared with a similar group who did not participate in the instructional program. And psychologists Perry London and David Engstrom of the University of California at Irvine have trained patients with low back pain to control their pain through coping strategies such as relaxation, deep breathing, and use of imagery.

Your body has very real, very profound healing power within. The primary component of this healing power is awareness, and awareness can be achieved by anybody. I, for instance, was not aware of spirituality in medicine until I had been practicing for many years. Now I see that most of our problems originate in our minds, that most of our diseases are diseases of self, brought on by the self. When I say that disease is a self-induced experience, I mean that it's a result of a maladjustment to life or life situations, or to an inordinate amount of stress or an inappropriate diet. But ultimately the origin of the disease is the mind.

That's why treating illness medically alone doesn't heal. It's only a temporary solution to the physical manifestation of the problem. True healing requires something more.

I have seen people heal themselves from obesity, from smoking, and from high blood pressure, all without taking drugs. The studies of Dr. Dean Ornish have shown significant improvement in coronary artery disease with just diet, exercise, meditation, and support.

These facts have opened up my mind to the idea that we all have the power to heal ourselves. The only problem is that that power can remain unused for our entire lives if we don't become aware of it. So the key to creating a healing personality is evoking your ability to heal yourself.

How can you evoke that healing power? First, and most important, be aware that it exists. Open yourself up to the spiritual dimension of yourself, the dimension that is always free from disease. Open yourself to becoming a self-healer; be aware of your body and its true needs.

Second, believe that you can get better. In two separate studies, psychologists Suzanna Kobasa and Salvatore Maddi of the University of Chicago demonstrated that a positive appraisal of control is the activator that triggers our internal healing mechanisms and keeps our immune systems from turning against us. In the first study, the team evaluated 200 Bell Telephone executives with high stress in their lives. Half the volunteers reported multiple symptoms of illness, while the others described themselves as healthy. The healthy group tested as having a positive appraisal of control during stress; they reported considering change a normal part of life and were able to control their reactions to problems. In the second study, 100 gynecology outpatients with high stress levels were compared. The forty women with few symptoms also displayed a greater sense of control, exemplified by a commitment to self, family, and work, and a stronger sense of challenge as compared with the group with more severe symptoms.

Faith and a sense of connection also help to activate the healer within. In a study of 212 patients who underwent coronary bypass or aortic valve replacement operations, R. Thomas Oxmanon, a psychiatrist, reported in *Internal Medicine News* of July 1993 that the risk of death after heart surgery rises for patients with no religious beliefs. Numerous other studies have demonstrated that isolation from social or community groups carries an increased risk of mortality.

WRITING YOUR OWN SCRIPT

Whether you are currently healthy, already have heart disease, or even have had a heart attack, you can begin to write your own script for a healthy heart right now.

But before writing any script, it is important to set the stage. In this case, setting the stage means making sure that you have done everything possible to evaluate the present condition of your heart and circulatory system. That should include a visit to your physician or cardiologist to have a thorough checkup, especially if you haven't had one recently.

The doctor will advise you to take a number of tests, particularly if any abnormalities show up. After a complete physical examination, your doctor may also order an electrocardiogram (ECG). In this test, electrodes are placed on the skin of your chest and hooked up to a machine that records your heartbeats. Unfortunately, the resting ECG is normal in over 50 percent of patients who may have coronary disease.

To increase the sensitivity of the ECG, we can perform an exercise test. This time you will walk on a treadmill while your blood pressure and heart are monitored. Any irregularities of your heartbeat and whether the cardiogram changes during exertion can be observed: This is relevant because we can detect changes in the ECG that are not accompanied by pain. It shows if your blood pressure goes higher than it should for the degree of exercise you are doing, which, of course, you would be unaware of, and most important, it reveals how you perform. The longer you are able to walk on the treadmill, the more faith the doctor will have in the strength of your heart muscle.

If abnormalities are detected in the treadmill test, another test, called thallium stress, is performed. In this test you walk on the treadmill as before while a radioisotope that has a special affinity for the heart is injected into a vein in your arm. Your heart is then monitored through an X-ray machine to show either a uniform distribution of the radioisotope or areas that are deprived of blood flow.

If all of the above tests are abnormal, the final test is the coronary angiography, in which your coronary arteries are examined with X-ray techniques. This procedure is done when you are awake, lying on a special X-ray table. Local anesthesia is applied to your arm or groin, and a thin polyethylene tube called a catheter is inserted and advanced to the coronary arteries. A radiopaque liquid is injected, and pictures are taken at a speed of thirty frames a second. When the procedure is completed, the catheter is removed and the artery repaired. You rest for seven or eight hours and then are able gradually to resume your regular activities.

This is an extremely important test because it reveals any area of coronary narrowing, blockage, or spasm and indicates if you are a candidate for surgery or other therapeutic measures.

Once you have determined your current condition, have worked with your doctor to evaluate any risk factors, and have assessed the health of your other body organs, it is time to add to your script the other elements of a healthy heart. All of these will be explored in detail in the following chapters.

MAKING A CONTRACT WITH YOUR HEART

Think back to the seven keys for a healthy heart in Chapter 2. Chances are you are already following some of the suggestions and need to work on others. I realize that starting anything new, even something so positive as a healthy lifestyle, can seem overwhelming. I read somewhere that we see obstacles when we have lost sight of our goals. This is important to remember if you are feeling overwhelmed.

You should keep in mind that having a healthy heart is your goal—and the first step toward achieving this goal is to be committed to it. Think of it as a personal contract that you are making with your heart. If it is easier, you can even write down a specific contract stating that you promise yourself to take the best possible care of your heart and then establish specific goals.

But don't make the goals too grandiose. You can't promise that you will immediately give up all bad habits, lose fifty pounds, and take up swimming all at once. That doesn't work. Instead, learn to divide the goal into small parts. For example, if your goal is to begin a walking program, your first minigoal might be to buy a pair of gym shoes. Your second minigoal could be choosing which part of the day you would like to dedicate to this special activity, and then the third would be to begin to do it on a regular basis. So, step by step, you will achieve what you have planned.

Each person's contract is naturally going to be a little different. For example, if you would like to lose weight, you could write in the contract that in six months you would like to weigh so much, or that in six months you'd like to be able to walk a certain distance comfortably.

The key is that you have specific and realistic goals in mind.

When we create possibilities and objectives for the future, we make them part of the present in the sense that it is today that we start pursuing them. Beginning, it has been said, is winning. If you never start, you will never win.

In addition to writing a plan and drawing up a contract, it can be very helpful to start visualizing yourself as having already achieved your goals. I'll have more to say about visualization later.

It may seem strange to think of making a contract with your heart, but your heart is a part of you, and the more you think about it and communicate with it, the more responsive it will be. Chet, a fifty-three-year-old doctor, had a heart attack and all at once was faced with mortality. He put it like this, "I suddenly faced a timetable which before then I never had to face because I was going to live some more in the distant future—not forever, but I didn't have to put a time limit on it. And then, all of a sudden, I was faced with it and had to make plans for it. I had this feeling of fragility about my existence.

"For me, it lasted about four weeks. At the end of that time I said to myself, 'If this is life, you may as well die because you're not doing anything.' So then I decided I was going to live. I started talking to my heart. I said, 'You either keep up with me, or, if you don't, we'll both die together.' It was a conscious decision. That's when I started cardiac rehab and I started walking. I went through six weeks of cardiac rehab and continued with exercise."

So Chet made the deal with his heart, and within a few months he was back doing what he had done before the heart attack.

WHAT TO SAY WHEN YOU
TALK TO YOURSELF

I am thoroughly convinced that the greatest sources of stress in life are the conversations we have with ourselves. These inner dialogues are too often negative and self-destructive. They often go something like this: "When are you going to learn? Oh, no, you did it again!"

We criticize ourselves, we put ourselves down. We reserve for ourselves treatment that we may have received in childhood, often undeservedly. But regardless of where such negative remarks come from, we need to get rid of them. After all, what do we get at the end of our criticism? What do we get from putting ourselves down? Nothing except a feeling of low self-esteem and inadequacy.

The good news is that we don't have to continue this way of thinking. To stop, first realize that you are the only thinker in your mind. That may sound obvious or even silly, but it's true. If you are the only person who is thinking, then you can choose unilaterally what to think. Instead of continuing with a cascade of negative self-talk, you can consciously choose positive self-talk.

Now when I talk to myself I watch my language. I realize that I have to stop criticizing myself and begin using affirmative words. I choose to love and appreciate myself. I have changed my thoughts. When I do have a negative experience, I ask myself how I can learn something from it instead of blame myself for it. I turn it around to my advantage.

Negative self-talk can be even more destructive if you already have heart disease or fear of heart disease. For instance, suppose you have a chest pain. Now your thoughts can heighten the seriousness of this pain to the point where it becomes immobilizing. It can frighten you terribly. You may not know what to do; doubt and anxiety may prevent you from thinking clearly. You can control this feeling by talking to yourself in a positive way. For example, if you are having mild, exercise-induced angina, tell yourself that all you are having is angina, not a heart attack. Angina is the way your heart talks to you, and it is telling you to slow down and rest.

Furthermore, if you keep in mind disease instead of health, if you continue to see yourself as a sick person instead of a healthy person with a heart problem, if you focus on prolonging life instead of living life, this limited vision will hurt your health.

Don't let this happen to you. Remember that how healthy you are is much more important than how sick you are. A healthy heart is not one that is physically perfect but one that is at peace.

Positive Self-talk for Chest Pain/Angina

Effective Talk	*Negative Talk*
My heart is talking to me.	This pain frightens me.
I know what to do.	I am powerless.
If I stop and relax, the pain will go away.	I'm getting nervous, anxious, short of breath.
If I take care of the pain, I am in control.	I am afraid to die.
Getting nervous and fearful does not help.	I'm out of control.
I had pain other times and I know what to do.	The pain means a heart attack.
I'm now calm and confident.	I don't know what is going to happen.

HEARTSKILL 3: SENDING HEALING ENERGY TO YOUR HEART

Your heart is the site of love. Your heart symbolizes the temple of your soul. Your heart is the most intimate part of you. Your heart is the source of life. When your heart stops, your life stops. With all this in mind, don't you think you should become more aware of this divine organ? You can do so by listening to it with a stethoscope and paying attention to the beautiful rhythmic sound that it produces.

As you learn the rhythm of your heart, you can send healing energy to it to keep it healthful and strong.

If you already have heart disease, you can help the recovery process by visualizing your heart as perfect. To do this, draw a picture of a healthy heart. Draw it free from disease or blemish or blockage. Think about that image; imagine that it is the picture of the heart beating within your chest.

Use the following meditation once a day to send more healing energy to your heart. First, tape the message in a slow, calm voice. Then find a comfortable chair, sit, close your eyes, and relax your muscles. When you feel thoroughly relaxed, play the tape to yourself.

MEDITATION FOR HEALING

Close your eyes and relax. Now visualize your heart as a powerful, divine organ. Imagine a light that permeates your body, healing every cell and specifically your heart. Visualize your heart beating regularly and perfectly. Visualize the strength of the heart muscle as it continues to beat within your chest.

Form a mental image of the arteries that surround your heart like a crown. See them with smooth walls, free from any disease as they deliver an abundant flow of blood. See the blood, in turn, rich in oxygen and nutrients necessary for perfect heart function. The light enters the heart and pulsates with it. See waves of healing light shining from the heart and bathing every cell in your body.

Your heart is the center of your spirit. Your heart is the center of love.

Chapter Six

THE FRIENDSHIP FACTOR

---

*Life is an island in an ocean
of loneliness.*
—Kahlil Gibran

The literature of psychoneuroimmunology is filled with clinical proof of the direct physical benefits of social support to patients. This effect is manifested even if the support is no more than a momentarily held hand, a pat on the arm, or a warm smile.

I remember Sara, who had been in a coma for days. Her eyes were closed, and she appeared to be locked into her own little world. Her vital signs were poor; her blood pressure was low. Yet when her family walked into the room her blood pressure rose to normal. The positive effect of their presence on her brain and her body chemistry was clear and evident.

A sense of support, or lack of it, greatly influences our view of life and is probably the major factor in our appraisals of our own life's meaning and value. Marian Diamond of the University of California at Berkeley has demonstrated over the past thirty years that the brain is adaptable and can be changed by our perceptions. When people find the elements in their lives interesting, enriching, attractive—in other words, when they have positive stimulation as opposed to loneliness and isolation—the neurons in the cortex apparently enlarge. Increased social contact has also been found to strengthen the immune system, while loss of support weakens it.

The *American Journal of Epidemiology* reported a study of a population survey that established a direct association between social networks and mortality. Subjects who had more social and community ties were more likely to live longer. Furthermore, a recent University of Minnesota study among bone marrow transplant patients showed that those who had strong emotional support from their families or friends had a 54 percent survival rate during the two-year follow-up. For those with little social support, the two-year survival rate was only 20 percent.

Researchers have also shown that social interaction has a strong effect on the health of the heart and circulatory system. Dr. Stephen Manuck, studying monkeys under stressful social conditions, found that the more gregarious a monkey is, the less likely it is to develop heart disease. In a study published in *The Annals of Internal Medicine*, researchers found that elderly men and women who had two or more sources of emotional support lived measurably longer after a heart attack than those with no support. It seems no matter what the illness, social isolation shortens patients' life spans.

A sense of social support is crucial to the recovery of heart patients. Heart disease is a disease of loneliness and the inability to share oneself. It's a disease of isolation. Thus, to achieve a complete cure, it is necessary to reestablish connections with others and with oneself.

The healing mechanism that social support provides isn't yet known. It may be, as Blair Justice, author of *Who Gets Sick*, points out, that when we maintain a sense of support and control in life we are inducing our neuroregulators to trigger the body's self-healing mechanisms. In this view the body reads messages of "no support" and "no control" as signals to shut down. Isolation is the perfect example of "no support" and the very opposite of an experience of meaning or purpose that necessarily involves feelings of connectedness with other people.

I think of Anna, an elderly patient whom I visited in the hospital. She has not only advanced heart disease but also cancer spread throughout her body. That day she was lying down, receiving oxygen through a nasal tube. She replied to my greeting with a beatific smile.

How could this sick woman manage such a beautiful smile? The answer was all around her. Next to her and embracing her was one of her sons. In the same room was another son, two sisters-in-law, and a five-year-old child. They were all happy and relaxed.

I suddenly realized that the strength that enabled Anna to continue came from the feeling that her family gave to her of being loved and wanted. Medications play only a part in the healing process. Love is keeping Anna alive and comfortable. I told her so, and she nodded in agreement. As I was leaving, I kissed her. She smiled, saying, *"Que Dios le proteja."*

We were sharing the same love.

SEXUAL INTIMACY: THE HEALING TOUCH

Following a heart attack, some patients lose confidence in themselves from a fear of loss of attractiveness, or even a fear of death. As a result, they may hesitate or even refuse to resume sexual relations with a spouse. Yet there is probably no time when the reassurance and sharing of sexual intimacy is more important.

The truth is that the desire for sex is a basic human need not limited to healthy people. If you have a heart problem, you still have sexual impulses, and denying or ignoring them may be a source of additional stress. What more beautiful way than the intimacy of sex to touch another and be touched in return? I call it the healing touch.

Yet for some recovering heart patients, psychological factors interfere with—and prevent—the resumption of sexual activity. In addition to the fears I just mentioned, a common fear is that of performance. You may feel that you won't be as good a lover as you were before the heart attack or surgery. Or you may be depressed because of what has happened to you and its reminder of your mortality.

I understand your concerns. After a heart attack you are frightened, and reasonably so. I want to reassure you that this concern is perfectly normal. I also want to help put those fears to rest and assure you that there is no reason to give up your normal sex life.

Let me tell you about the changes that take place in your body during sex. The blood pressure and heart rate rise, breathing becomes faster, the skin gets flushed because of the increase in blood flow. As you get more excited, tension builds up; it is then released during orgasm. Gradually the blood pressure, heart rate, and breathing return to normal.

Now you may think this all sounds very strenuous, but in fact the physical energy spent during sexual activity is equivalent to walking briskly up two flights of stairs. Precisely because of this element of exercise, sex may be good for you—certainly better than a strong emotion that has no release.

It's true that there is a very small risk of heart attack during sexual activity, but this risk is almost exclusively confined to people making love with someone other than their regular, legitimate partners. Death during sexual activity is very rare. A study by M. Ueno, reported in *The Japanese Journal of Legal Medicine* in 1963, found that coital death accounted for only 0.6 percent of sudden deaths in males, and that in most cases the man was with someone other than his wife. Furthermore, the men were an average of thirteen years older than their female companions, and one-third were intoxicated.

So there is really no reason to let fear prevent you from resuming your normal sexual activity after your diagnosis of heart problems or surgery. How soon you can engage in sex varies from person to person, but most experts advise that you are well enough to resume sexual activity when you can climb two flights of stairs. The majority of men and women do resume sex within a few weeks after a heart attack. If you are afraid to resume sex or don't know if you are well enough, discuss the matter with your physician and ask for an exercise test. This way your tolerance for exertion can be determined without your being put in any danger.

Once you are confident that you can resume your regular sexual activities, remember that your sexual drive may be affected by medications you are taking. It's important to discuss any such potential problems with your physician. Remember also that you don't need to set any records, especially right away. Sexual activity, like all other activities, should be resumed gradually. I advise my patients to think of the romantic aspects of sex. Begin with caressing, holding, kissing, and hugging.

Beyond that, it's up to you and your partner. The American Heart Association (AHA) recommends that the best times for sex while you are recovering are in the morning, after resting, and before taking medications. The exception to the no-medication guideline is that if you are taking nitroglycerine for angina it can be helpful to take it before sexual activity, especially if you are afraid of chest pains.

Three-fourths of all heart surgery patients are able to return to the frequency of intercourse and positions during sexual activity that they had before surgery. For some, a change of position may be necessary; for instance, you should avoid positions that put pressure on the chest. The AHA also recommends waiting for at least three hours after a meal before having sex, because during digestion the body's blood supply is concentrated in the intestines, making less of it available to the heart.

The most important point to remember about sexual relations is that if you are fortunate enough to have a partner, you must be open and sincere and find solutions to your worries and problems together. If you avoid sex out of fear of making your heart condition worse or causing another attack, you may be adding a greater source of stress to your system than the sex itself would. Also remember that there is a big difference between having sex and making love. To be touched and loved is a fundamental human need, and satisfying that need is indispensable.

KEEPING YOUR LOVED ONES HEALTHY AND LETTING THEM KEEP YOU HEALTHY

Shortly before going to the cath lab for an emergency coronary angioplasty, Alberta, an eighty-four-year-old lady with gray hair, blue eyes, and a broad smile, jokingly told me that she had already survived four doctors. When I asked her how she had managed this feat, she laughed. "Why," she said, "I don't have time to get sick. I have to take care of my four daughters and all of their children."

Alberta was the living embodiment of the truth that our families can be our deepest source of support—whether they take care of us or we take care of them. At the same time, every member of the family is affected if one of them has heart disease. The other family members can become anxious and fearful, especially when the person with heart disease is the mother or father.

If a parent must stop working temporarily or permanently because of illness, the stress on the family is even worse. In addition to the humiliation the parent feels at having to discontinue providing financial support, he or she also can become paralyzed with concern about the future. The spouse too will usually become fearful, though he or she may not express those fears openly.

The solution to many problems caused by the heart disease of one member of the family is open communication among all, especially between the patient and the spouse. If the children are old enough, include them too. Let them feel that they are a part of all conferences and decisions that are made. Reassure them that you will recover, and that from now on you will take better care of yourself. At the same time, ask for their support in helping you to maintain a new, healthy schedule, for instance, or simply in working toward recovery. I often recommend that family members hug, touch, and hold each other and the patient as much as possible. I also suggest saying "I love you" and letting the patient know how vital he or she is to the family's well-being.

Although everyone in the family must remain aware of the heart problem and any potential for recurrence, it is also important not to let the heart problem dominate family life. As a patient you must remember that your heart condition is only one part of your life. I want to add that "family" does not necessarily mean only blood family or family by marriage. Anyone with whom you have a close, ongoing relationship can be considered a part of your family in this context.

A Spiritual Giant

I will never forget Steve, perhaps the most memorable of my exceptional heart patients. A tall, blue-eyed ex-Marine, Steve conveyed a sense of strength, power, and confidence to everyone who met him. At the age of fifty, after two open-heart surgeries, Steve developed lung cancer. He survived for five years, but then the cancer returned, and at last the decision was made to allow him to go home and die among the people he loved.

When I visited him at home, he was lying in a hospital bed in the living room, surrounded by flowers and the pictures of his children. His bed looked out on the garden. Despite his emaciated, exhausted appearance, he greeted me warmly. I checked his blood pressure and his lungs. I felt we were communing even though he was too weak to talk.

His wife told me that he'd had a beautiful afternoon conversing with his daughter. They both sat looking out at the garden full of flowers and listening to birds singing. As I left, I felt that he was surrounded by love.

In the middle of the night I received a phone call from his wife: It was over. His brave Marine heart had finally given up. At his funeral, as in life, he was surrounded by those who had loved him and symbols of the things that had been most meaningful in his life. There were a multitude of people I didn't recognize, along with flowers and flags. Lying peacefully, Steve was dressed smartly in a suit and tie. In the coffin with him were pictures of his children and grandchildren, of himself and his wife. His family had re-created the atmosphere of home for him in his coffin. I had never seen anything like this in the twenty-five years I have lived in the United States.

I still carry with me the card Steve gave me, which said, "To Dr. B. Cortis. To my doctor. To my friend. To the person I love like a brother."

JOINING OR STARTING YOUR OWN SUPPORT GROUP

Support groups of all sorts have been springing up around the country. This is natural because like-minded people who have been through similar difficulties or who have similar health problems can help one another.

After thirty years of cardiology practice, I realized that teaching people how to be healthy was more fulfilling than identifying disease. As a result, I created in my office a large conference room where I meet periodically with patients to discuss preventive medicine. I explain the value of diagnostic tests, the harmful effects of stress—in short, all the things I am sharing with you in this book. But there is one thing this book cannot do: share back, as my patients and I do when we gather to talk about our feelings and life experiences.

The results of these meetings have been gratifying, both to me and to the patients who attend them. The patients have different goals. Some lost weight, others cut down on the number of medications they took, some stopped smoking. In distinct ways they all became more responsible for their own health.

When I see these results, I feel that I am truly fulfilling my role as a physician-teacher by empowering my patients and enabling them to become responsible and healthy. In creating this support group, my patients and I are able to manifest our humanity fully. We totally accept one another and share unconditional caring for one another in these sessions. One patient recently told me, "I like you as a physician, but even more as a person." I feel the same way about them. I value them as patients, but I love them as people. I have discovered the joy of deeper patient-physician relationships and achieved a better understanding of myself and others through them.

In light of the value I have found and seen others enjoy in such sharing groups, I urge you to try to find one of your own. There are a growing number of cardiac support groups all over the country. These groups usually meet in hospitals or in private institutions where cardiac patients can gather not only to discuss common problems but to celebrate when one of them has surgery, comes back from surgery, or is recovering. They notify members when someone is ill or dying so that each person has visitors up until the very end.

Your own doctor, local hospital, or Y probably can provide

you with a list of local support groups. Some combine exercise and support, others merely meet for discussions. Shop around and find which group is best for you. If you are unable to find a local group, start your own. Put a notice up on the bulletin board in your doctor's office, the hospital, the local Y, or even the supermarket. Starting a group is relatively easy; all that is needed is a meeting place. Members can share this responsibility by having meetings at one another's houses.

Despite all my positive feelings about cardiac support groups, I do have one suggestion on how to improve them. Members of these groups are generally those who share the same health experiences. I would like to see more such support groups opened up to the general public, so that everybody has access to this treasure of knowledge and experience and more people may learn how to avoid becoming patients.

VOLUNTEERING FOR BETTER HEALTH

Just as contact with friends, family, and colleagues can have a positive impact on health and well-being, altruistic actions can free people from isolation and loneliness. An excellent way to increase your social contacts while doing something positive for the world is to volunteer. Schools, charities, and churches all need willing volunteers. If you are physically limited, perhaps you can answer phones or address envelopes.

Sheila, a hospital volunteer I know, helps stroke victims. Although she herself has been left handicapped by a stroke and has partial paralysis on her left side, she always greets me with a warm smile, asking, "How do you feel today?" and waves her right hand in a friendly way. Her eyes express a deep sense of purpose, the joy of caring for others unconditionally.

Another volunteer I know, Seymour, works up to five days a week in a local hospital, greeting patients' families and directing them to their loved ones' rooms. Though he is in ill health himself, Seymour seldom misses a day at work—he has told me he feels working keeps him young.

Volunteers can be of all ages. My daughter, Veronica, works as a volunteer in the emergency room at Loyola University. "I love to help other people," she told me the other day. Her most fulfilling moments have come when she has been able to hold the hand of a frightened child or reassure a recent widow.

Perhaps the day is not so far off when a doctor's prescription will read, "For loneliness, volunteer two evenings at the community food bank."

HEARTSKILL 4: MAPPING YOUR
SOCIAL SUPPORT SYSTEM

I hope the material in this chapter has convinced you of the importance of social support in your life. This support enables us to share feelings and emotions, to overcome isolation. Through our individual support systems we learn to face problems and worries by enriching ourselves with others' experiences.

However you choose to do it, sharing information and support is invaluable. It will help you learn more about your disease and provide you with a group of people with whom you can identify. It is rewarding to know others who understand and accept us and who share similar concerns. When we can interact with like-minded people, our problems do not cause isolation and separation and we can deal with each crisis more easily.

How strong is your social support system? To answer this question you must look first at the most important part of your system: you. Begin by spending time alone and focusing on discovering your true self. Be aware of the conversations you have with yourself, and try to discontinue those that are negative and disempowering. The other members of your group include your family, friends, and perhaps co-workers. Ideally all these people accept, respect, and appreciate you just the way you are. The knowledge that these are people who love and care about you nurtures you emotionally and spiritually. As you talk to your friends about your problems, you are also able to listen to what's troubling them. This act of sharing gives you the opportunity to evaluate your thoughts and feelings objectively.

The following inventory will help you find where your own support is, or could be. Grab a pencil and quickly jot down the answers to the following questions:

- Who would listen to me, no matter what?
- Who would lend me money?
- Who would come in the middle of the night?
- Who notices how my health is?
- Who notices how my projects are going?
- Who do I think of calling when I want to have fun?
- If I received some wonderful, unexpected news that had to be kept secret for a time, who would I tell anyway?

If you thought of anyone who would come in the middle of the night, you have support; the rest is gravy.

If you aren't happy with all your answers, you need to make an effort to expand your social support base. Start by finding people who like what you like. They are already in the places and doing the things that make you feel happy. If you like to build model airplanes, these people can be found at model airplane clubs. If you are a bridge player, they are down at the local duplicate game. I have found many of my support people at self-development programs, where I like to spend my free time.

Remember that if you find people through activities you enjoy, these things make them happy, too, so you already have a bond even though you may not have met yet. Start building your support group indirectly by getting involved in activities you like in the place that feels best to you. Don't worry if you don't ever have a list of friends a mile long. Many people find a few really dependable friends are enough support. Leave room in your life to add others, but take the initiative. Make the first move to get to know people, and you'll find that the best way to find a friend is to be one.

Chapter Seven

OPENING YOUR HEART

TO YOURSELF

Great peace have they which love.
—Psalms

There are patients, believe it or not, who are actually happy to have a heart attack. A few days ago a patient told me that now that he's had a heart attack he has a sense of relief because he finally *has* to do the things he knows he needs to do, such as exercise, eat sensibly, and rest. "Before the heart attack," he told me, "I didn't *have* to do them, and since I didn't have to, I didn't. I always found excuses, like not enough time, or that they weren't really that important. But now that I have to do them, I feel free. I feel for the first time I can live my life."

He was smiling when he said these words, but I could see that he meant them. For the first time in his life, he was putting himself first.

The subject of this chapter may sound strange to you or make you feel uncomfortable. It is self-love, literally loving and caring for yourself. Although love of self is important to everyone, it is especially important to heart patients.

When I first started thinking about self-love, a funny question occurred to me. How do I know that I love myself? It took me several minutes to come up with two answers. The first was that I like to take care of my body. The second has to do with vanity. I like to dress well, so I concluded that if I take the time, money, and effort to do this, I must love myself. Then more and more answers came: I like my own company, I love my sense of humor and my creativity, I feel that I am divinely guided. I know I deserve my love because I am kind, sensitive, open-minded, and loving. I love the spirit of God within me.

Now all of this may sound self-centered, but in reality it is self-protective. The more you love yourself, the better you will take care of yourself and the healthier you will be. Nobody would doubt that being told by others that we are lovable is important to our health and well-being. I believe that it is just as important that we say it to ourselves, that we constantly express our love and in so doing reinforce the idea that we are creatures of love and emotion as well as thinking, rational beings.

I remember a patient, Jay, who had a severe heart attack in his early fifties. Before the attack he had been a professor, an intellectual who had developed only his mind and not taken care of his body or his spirit. After the heart attack he undertook a rigorous program of rehabilitation and completely changed his life orientation. "Now I live in my heart," Jay told me. "I have discovered that any and all healing takes place completely in the heart. People who reside in the mind do not live in the moment and are not capable of real, deep intimacy with themselves or with another human being."

I congratulated Jay on this insight, but he had more. "In my first life," he said, referring to the time before his heart attack, "I cared about looking good and performing for others. But now I know that I deserve to have my own life support me, that I deserve to protect myself and love myself. I know now that my life contributed to my needing the heart operation well beyond the genetic considerations."

THE VALUE OF SELF-ESTEEM

As you can see from Jay's story, loving yourself doesn't have to mean self-indulgence. Nor does it just mean appreciating your good points. It also means accepting your limitations. All of these are a part of something called self-esteem, which is the opinion we have of ourselves. Our self-esteem is shaped by many factors, including how we were treated as children and all of our past victories and so-called failures.

Unfortunately, many of us do not have true self-esteem. Instead we have a self-image that is distorted by experiences in childhood. For example, did anyone ever tell you, "You are not good enough for X" or "Don't do Y"? When you repeatedly hear such messages at the age of five or six, you come to believe them and grow up with the idea that you are not good in a particular field or that you aren't allowed to do certain things. Of course most of these negative messages were a result of our parents' attempts to protect us, but they can be a source of false limitations throughout life.

I remember once when I was a small boy I sang a bawdy song that someone had taught me. I repeated it to my family, not understanding the words, and was punished. As a result, I stopped singing.

The consequence of listening to such negative messages is that we tend to behave according to who we think we are instead of who we really are. To learn to love the true us we must learn to accept ourselves, warts and all. You can't like the left side of your face, after all, and hate the right side. You can't like yourself from the belly button up and hate yourself from the belly button down. Learning to accept yourself is the best way to improve your self-esteem.

Self-esteem, according to Nathaniel Branden, author of *Psychology of Self-esteem*, is a combination of two components, self-confidence and self-respect. Self-confidence is the ability to think, to judge, to recognize and be able to correct mistakes. You are self-confident when you feel you can handle a situation. Self-respect, on the other hand, is a sense of worthiness. Both of these need to come from within.

Unfortunately, many of us let our self-esteem depend too much on factors beyond our control. Physicians are an example of this. You see, as a result of how we are trained, we feel guilt when anything negative happens to a patient. I've talked to plenty of other surgeons, and we all agree, when a patient dies we suffer terribly. But by doing this we are really hurting ourselves, because we are basing our self-esteem on factors we can't control. I'll give you an example. One day I happened to be in the hospital when a man went into cardiac arrest and I resuscitated him. I immediately began mouth to mouth and did everything I could to bring him back. When he regained consciousness he opened his eyes, then later looked straight at me and said, "I wanted to die."

I was shocked. I didn't know what to think. All I could say was "I didn't know that." I spoke to his family, and we transferred him from the coronary care unit to another department, where he gradually got his wish.

I felt terrible—both because I had gone against his wishes, without even knowing them, and because he had died. What the experience taught me was that, even if you're doing your best, you can still be wrong. You may be acting against the wishes of the person you are trying to help. Maybe he wants to be sick, or maybe she thinks she has an incurable disease, or for whatever reason maybe he even wants to die. As simple as this is to say and comprehend, it still hurts when a patient dies.

The point here is that I can't let such an incident damage my own self-love, my self-esteem.

A POSITIVE APPROACH TO
NEGATIVE EMOTIONS

Of course we all have areas in our lives that we consider less than ideal and often judge from these that we are unlovable. But this is no reason to condemn ourselves. Remember that the more you accept yourself the easier it is to accept other people and the easier it is for them to accept you.

One way to do this is to learn to recognize negative emotions, and then, instead of fighting them, replace them with positive ones. One of the worst things a heart patient can do is fight or resist these emotions. For example, suppose you hate the dark. Fighting it would be useless. But recognizing it for what it is— the absence of light—gives you the key to overcoming the problem. All you have to do is turn on a light . . . and the darkness vanishes!

In the same way, when you recognize a negative emotion— say fear—analyze it but don't fight it. Then try to replace it with a more positive emotion. For example, suppose you are afraid of a heart attack. Instead of sitting and stewing about it, which can make your condition worse, take some positive steps. Start an exercise program or cut back on the fat in your diet. At the same time, replace your negative thought of a sick heart with a positive thought of a healthy heart. The importance of replacing the old idea is that it opens the door to new possibilities of thought and action.

Another way to deal with negative thoughts and emotions is to realize that some of the things we think we believe are not our own thoughts and emotions at all. In a way we inherited them. These thoughts started out in another person's mind, maybe a parent, or teacher, or some authority figure seen on TV. For example, I once had a patient who was convinced that she had serious heart disease. This woman was in her sixties, overweight, inactive, and depressed, and her treadmill test was abnormal. But when the angiogram showed mild coronary disease, she changed her life completely. She became joyful, lost weight, and began to exercise regularly. In short, she began to live her life fully.

So be aware of your thoughts and first distinguish what is negative from what is positive and worthwhile. Then try to identify and get rid of any thoughts that don't belong to you.

LETTING GO OF TYPE A BEHAVIOR

The following quotation is from an article about physicians with heart disease: "The outstanding feature was the incessant treadmill of practice. Every one of these men had an additional factor, worry; in not a single case under fifty years of age was this feature absent."

Does this description sound familiar? It could apply to many of us, not just physicians. To me, the interesting thing about this paragraph is that it was published in 1924, describing a group of physicians who were sick in 1910. Thirty years later, Flanders Dunbar described patients with coronary artery disease: "They are compulsive, have a tendency to work long hours and not take vacations, a tendency to seize authority; dislike of sharing responsibility. . ."

Today such people would be described as Type A personalities, and unfortunately they still seem to get more than their share of heart disease. Although everyone is different, the Type A person is involved in a chronic struggle to achieve more and more in less and less time. Type A behavior can cause physical damage in several ways. It can increase cholesterol level, blood pressure, and the likelihood of developing diabetes. Not surprisingly, Type A people are often cigarette smokers, which only makes their health problems worse.

Where does Type A behavior come from? Usually there are many factors, one of the most powerful of which is the pressure to compete. We do live in a competitive world, but for some of us it seems that everything must be part of a contest. "I must make more money, I must prove I am the best salesman, husband, father. . . ." Not all Type A behavior is detrimental. Competition in itself can be constructive. But the anger and hostility that often accompany extreme competitiveness have been linked with an increased risk of heart attack.

Unfortunately, the culture itself encourages this destructive behavior with its materialistic assumption that nothing counts unless it can be counted. We have one car, but that's not enough, we need two cars, three cars. We need one TV for each child. This is, in essence, a disease of more. I hope you can see that it is a trap, and that there is no reason to be constantly in competition with anyone, least of all yourself.

Another source of Type A behavior is the modern trend to reduce men and women to numbers and standardize them. We are not numbers. Each of us is an individual, a unique person with divine qualities. But in order to take advantage of them, we must become aware of them.

Finding the Time to Find Yourself

Perhaps the biggest contributor to Type A behavior is time pressure. It seems that these days everything must be done fast, instantly. We have instant coffee, Instant Breakfast, instant news summaries. This infatuation with *right now!* gives us a distorted perception of time. When we get sick, time seems to become even more important. How much time do I have? How much time is left? This panic reaction in relation to time can put more stress on someone who is already stressed by a heart attack.

It is important to ask ourselves what, really, is time? By definition it is the sequence of events. We use time to indicate that one occurrence happens after or before another. Time is just a frame of reference. But each of us perceives time differently. For some it seems to go fast; for others it seems to go slow. Circumstances can change our perception of time. People who are in pain often have a sense of time going very slowly, while pain medication can speed things up again. Even in day-to-day life our perception of time changes. When we are in a hurry, we are anxious; when we feel we have plenty of time, we are calm and relaxed. So much is based on our perception of time.

One of the best ways to begin to modify your own Type A behavior is to analyze, then change your perception of time. Paul Pearsall, author of *Super Immunity*, suggests that you use this exercise to get in touch with your idea of time: Sit in a comfortable chair and pretend that you are relaxing for one minute. Before you close your eyes, check the second hand on your watch, then wait for what seems like one minute. For some people one perceived minute may in reality be thirty seconds. For others it may be three minutes. The truth is, it matters how long a minute lasts for you. Ideally, you should decide to relax and, when you are relaxed, return to your activities refreshed and alert.

Another way to modify Type A behavior is to establish clear goals in life, or, if you don't like the word *goals*, priorities. I'm talking here of family goals, social goals, and personal goals. Think of the places you would like to see, people you would like to meet. Write your goals on paper; then devise a plan for reaching them and start to take action. As you do this, visualize yourself achieving your goals. Just the fact that you put them on paper gives them power; they become alive.

Control your work by learning the magic word *no*. When you are overwhelmed by work, when demands are excessive, save your life, save your health by saying "No." Control your work, rather than letting it control you.

I know this all sounds impossible, but I have had many, many patients who have completely changed their Type A behavior after being diagnosed with heart disease. Jay, whom I mentioned at the beginning of this chapter, admits that before his heart attack he was unaware of the way he acted. But after recovering he saw clearly what his life had been like. "I put such pressure on myself," he says now. "I did such a poor job at protecting my heart. I felt and absorbed everything. I was such a Type A personality, I felt betrayed by many people and also by myself. I thought I was a failure."

IDENTIFYING AND HEALING YOUR CHILDHOOD HURTS

The child that we once were stays with us forever. There is no one moment in our life when that child ends and the adult begins. This inner child, as it is called in popular psychology, is the part of ourselves that needs to be loved, to be acknowledged, to have fun. The adult, on the other hand, is the part that cares about financial commitments, responsibilities, deadlines, titles, and qualifications.

In a balanced life we should cultivate a harmonious relationship between the child and the adult within us. Each part must acknowledge the other's needs. This is especially important for cardiac patients, who often tend to ignore their own needs. Because of guilt from childhood, we may be denying ourselves the ability to celebrate our success or to relax and enjoy life.

But how do you know what your child's needs are? One way to find out is to sit in a comfortable chair, close your eyes, and visualize yourself at the age of four or five. Get a good picture in your mind, then listen to what that little child is saying to you.

If you have trouble imagining this tiny being, get a picture of yourself that was taken when you were very young. I did this and had it magnified by one of my patients. Then I looked straight into that little boy's eyes and saw who I was at that time. It was a beautiful feeling to get in touch with this inner child. Find out what your inner child needs and realize how you have grown away from the child within you as you have become a responsible adult.

When I began getting in touch with my inner child, I discovered some surprising facts. One of the memories that came back was that when I was very young I used to play with small snakes. I would hold them, scare people with them, and laugh. Today I would be extremely afraid even to touch a snake, although I know they are harmless. Somehow I've lost that spontaneity, curiosity, and child's courage. Another thing I used to do as a child was to tell jokes to adults and enjoy their laughter, yet now I am shy and sometimes afraid to talk in groups.

We all have stories like this, stories about how our inner child has been stifled, for whatever reason. This not only diminishes our joy of living but also leads to illness. I am convinced that losing touch with the child within is one of the factors behind heart disease. Getting in touch with your inner child is a way to understand and let go of those old hurts that have kept your childlike spirit repressed.

As you become a parent to yourself, remember that no one will ever know and love you as much as you can love yourself. Do not allow self-punishment to cause any more innocent tears. Instead, let the joy, spontaneity, and authenticity of your inner child come through and brighten every day of your life.

LEARNING TO FORGIVE

I often imagine some of my patients walking along holding a heavy object, like a chair. As they walk, they can choose which path to take, so they are seemingly free. However, in reality they are not free because they are carrying this extra weight, which becomes heavier and heavier with each step. It's only when they put down this load that they regain their freedom.

That imaginary weight is, of course, the burden of the past: resentments, angers, and guilts that we have heaped upon ourselves. To free ourselves from this oppression, we must learn to forgive ourselves and others. Leonard Laskow, in *Healing with Love*, writes that forgiving is *for giving* love to ourselves and others.

Forgiveness means letting go of the past. Whatever holds you to the past prevents you from truly experiencing the present. This notion is especially valid for some cardiac patients who have a tendency to see themselves as invalids. Naturally, this image prevents them from truly loving themselves.

Resentments are hostilities that we can't let go of; we keep dwelling on them in our minds. Letting go of these resentments is the same as forgiveness. How can you learn to let these go and to forgive yourself and others for past hurts? Here is a quick method suggested by Louise Hay: Make a list of the blessings you most want for yourself in life. Then pray for the person you resent to receive each of the blessings on your list. Do this once or twice a day for two weeks. At the end of that time, the resentful feelings will be either gone or greatly diminished.

HEARTSKILL 5: THOUGHT-LIFE INVENTORY

"Thoughts, beliefs, imaginations are not ephemeral abstractions but electrochemical events with physiological consequences," says Blair Justice. Justice is speaking here about a clinical study, but the same truth is found in the writings of the Greek philosopher Epictetus, who said, "Man is not disturbed by things, but by his opinion of things."

As we have seen, whether or not we are aware of them, our thoughts and emotions strongly affect our bodies, predisposing us to either illness or health. Emotions come from thoughts. So by controlling our thoughts we achieve control of our emotions. Obviously, the more control we can gain over these powerful rulers of our well-being the healthier we will be.

Bear in mind the things I have discussed about Type A behavior and its effects on the body. Investigators such as Redford Williams, chief of psychiatry at Duke University and author of *The Trusting Heart*, have demonstrated that a chronically hostile, cynical, or distrusting stance toward life is a contributor to heart disease.

The best way to avoid falling prey to these negative thoughts is to become aware of them. Ask yourself these questions: What feelings am I regularly feeding into my body's defenses that I am not aware of? What thoughts from childhood are affecting me that haven't yet caught up with my adult life?

Remember that, as in any activity, ways of thinking can become habits that we forget are a part of us. Still, these ways of thinking are influencing everything we do and say. What we focus our thoughts on becomes our experience. One way to become aware of these habits is to undertake a thought-life inventory to pinpoint the problem areas in our automatic thought processes and behavior.

Answer the following questions as honestly as you can; you don't have to share your answers with anyone. As you go through the inventory, become cognizant of what is being asked and how you answer. Remember that becoming aware of your own thinking is an acquired skill that takes practice.

When you evaluate your thought-life inventory, be on the lookout for this sort of frame of reference, which can have physically destructive consequences. Other damaging frames of reference, pointed out by author Joan Borysenko, include negative personal beliefs, rationalizations, shoulds, the need to be right, disillusionment, and despair.

Your Thought-Life Inventory

1. In casual conversation, how do you refer to yourself? (For instance, are you judgmental, saying, "I was a dummy," or perhaps self-congratulatory: "I really put one over on them.")

2. When you speak to yourself in your mind, how do you address and picture yourself? (List all names—for example, "You jerk!" "Sweetie," and so on.)

3. Which of these activities is common for you? Going to plays, concerts, exhibits, sports events; watching TV; seeing movies; reading; attending seminars or classes; listening to self-development tapes; participating in self-help or support groups.

4. What were your favorite books, movies, TV programs, and areas of interest as a child, teenager, and young adult, in middle life, and now?

5. Which five subject areas absorb the largest percentage of your conversation today? (You may have to ask your friends about this one.)

6. What offhand expressions are common in your speech? (Examples: "That's the way the cookie crumbles"; "Have a nice day"; and so on.)

7. Look around your living and work space. What images, posters, and sayings do you display for your own inspiration and enjoyment? (Sports heroes, religious figures, Garfield, and so on.)

8. If you could state your case to a powerful public figure, who would it be? What would your case be?

9. What sayings of parents or other important figures from your childhood or younger life do you still use in speaking to yourself or to others?

10. Who embodies the exact opposite of your ideas about personal life values, or how would you describe your exact opposite?

Evaluating Your Thought-Life Inventory

When you have completed the thought-life inventory, take a look at your answers and think about them. If you find thinking patterns that are not serving you well, you will probably also discover positive patterns that rightfully make you feel good.

For example, you may have observed that you refer to yourself as "dummy" or "stupid." Perhaps you noticed that you no longer or seldom enjoy the things you most enjoyed when you were younger. On the positive side, you may have discovered that you are interested in a wide variety of activities and subjects and that the objects you keep around you are cheerful and uplifting.

The positive aspects of your inventory point to directions in your development which, if you pursue them, will expand and invigorate other healthy thought patterns. These will increase your physical and mental well-being, and, now that you have identified negative patterns in your life, you can begin to eliminate them.

Chapter Eight

IDENTIFYING AND
HANDLING STRESS

In every real man a child is hidden that wants to play.
—Friedrich Nietzsche

W hat would you think if I told you that more than half of all your problems, both emotional and physical, came from the same source? Wouldn't you want to get rid of that cause as quickly as possible? Well, the truth is that approximately 75 percent of your problems do come from one cause—a cause with many roots—and that cause is stress. Stress affects your heart and your life. Unless you learn to control stress, it can control you.

What exactly is stress? Basically, it is the way the mind and body adapt to change. Physical stress, for example, would be a depletion of the body's resources caused by cold, illness, and exhaustion. But the most devastating, because it is the one we are least aware of, is psychological and emotional stress. There are several kinds of emotional stress, including stress brought on by family problems, social obligations, life changes, work, decision making, and phobias.

One reason that stress of any sort is so hard on our bodies and minds is that it takes away our sense of control over ourselves and/or our environment, which is one of the most basic human needs. If this need isn't met, we can become emotionally or physically unwell. A number of studies have demonstrated a link between stress and heart disease. In one experiment six groups of monkeys on a high-fat diet were put in cages of five monkeys each. As soon as the monkeys had established a pecking order, the members of three of the cages were shifted around, forcing them to establish a new order. Each month the monkeys in the experimental group were shifted, resulting in extreme stress as they had to keep beginning their battle for pecking order all over again. At the end of a year, the dominant monkeys in the experimental group had coronary arteries riddled with blockage. In the control group, on the other hand, the dominant monkeys had the lowest blockages. Evidently, the stress of continually proving their dominance had made the experimental monkeys ill.

Of course humans are different from monkeys, but apparently not so different in our reactions to stress. Several studies have shown a strong association between stress-related emotions, such as hostility, and coronary disease. Redford Williams, in *The Trusting Heart*, demonstrates a correlation between degree of hostility (cynicism, anger, aggressive behavior) and survival. In medical students followed for twenty-five years, the higher the hostility score, the higher the incidence of heart attacks and mortality. Similar death rates were found in 118 law school students followed for twenty-five years.

Another study, reported in *The New England Journal of Medicine*, told of a forty-four-year-old woman who had a heart attack immediately after learning about the suicide of her fourteen-year-old son.

Even seemingly unthreatening everyday events can produce a stress reaction. In a British study reported in *Lancet*, sixteen patients with coronary disease were hooked to ECG monitors and asked to perform relatively simple arithmetic problems. Although not all of the subjects experienced pain, all of their ECG monitors showed reduced blood supply to the heart.

TYPES OF STRESS

There are two basic types of stress: acute and chronic. Acute, or short-term, stress is prompted by an unexpected event that is perceived as a challenge to our sense of well-being and feeling that we are in control. This experience creates an alarm reaction characterized by fear, anxiety, sweating, and rapid heartbeat. Examples of short-term stress might include being involved in a car accident, hearing a fire alarm go off, or falling on an icy sidewalk. Our physical responses to these events are caused by hormonal reactions. The adrenal gland releases the hormone adrenaline. The sudden flood of adrenaline causes blood to be withdrawn from the skin and intestines and directed toward the muscles, preparing us to fight or flee. This reaction to stress is normal. It has evolved over the millennia, allowing our ancestors to survive in a very dangerous world, and it is still a helpful response in many situations.

The other type of stress, chronic stress, is much less adaptive, however, and can be harmful. Long-term stress occurs when we perceive a loss of control over ourselves or the environment that goes on. We experience a sense of failure and entrapment created by forces over which we have no control. Such strong feelings must go someplace. If we don't know what to do with the feelings and suppress them, their energy remains trapped in our bodies, like an electrical current that has been switched on.

This trapped energy is destructive to our hearts and our lives. The physiological responses to this include depression and increased secretion of cortisol, another hormone produced by the adrenal gland. Other changes include chronically elevated blood pressure; an increase in gastric secretions, which may lead to the development of ulcers; enhanced clotting agents in the blood; decreased production of sex hormones; augmented deposits of cholesterol in the arteries; and depression of the immune system.

Examples of situations leading to chronic stress include an unhappy marriage or job; money difficulties; chronic illness; and simply too many busy days with no time taken for rest. In many cases we bring about these situations with the demands we make on ourselves. I'm reminded of a colleague who recently died. As soon as I heard about his death, I started comparing his life with mine. It could happen to me, I thought. But then I recalled that he was a classic Type A personality working twenty-four hours a day. Not only that, but his life had changed in major ways before he got sick. His skills as a surgeon had slipped, he had had to change hospitals several times, and he must have suffered a terrible loss of self-esteem. All these factors make his death more understandable to me.

PERSONALITY TYPE AND STRESS

It's important to realize that stress itself is not the culprit in causing disease. It isn't something that assaults us from the outside, like a virus. Rather, stress is something that we create within ourselves. The real cause of stress-related illness lies in the way we perceive stress, and the way we react when we feel that we are losing control. Handling stress means controlling the anger, anxiety, and helplessness we experience in situations we perceive as stressful.

This is perhaps more important for heart patients than for other people. Dr. Robert Eliot, author of *Is It Worth Dying For?*, calls one in five healthy persons a "hot reactor." Hot reactors are people who have strong responses to stress and experience extreme rises in blood pressure when they feel out of control.

Perhaps not so strangely, heart disease itself is a significant source of stress. Probably no one has as much fear as a cardiac patient. There is the strong worry that every chest pain may be the beginning of a heart attack. There's the concern that exercise may precipitate angina; there's the fear of getting excited, the fear of a confrontation; there's the fear of premature death. Fear, fear, fear—there is no end to the fear and the stress it produces.

All these sources of stress, of course, affect people differently. An event may be particularly stressful for one person and pleasant for another, depending on a number of factors. According to Mark Tager and Stephen Willard, authors of *Transforming Stress into Power*, one way to handle stress is to learn which personality type you are. The *logical* type approaches life from a cause-and-effect perspective. These people focus on the here and now, and make decisions only when they feel they have enough facts. For the logical type of person, such as the fictional Mr. Spock on *Star Trek*, the greatest source of stress is illogical people—those who want things done yesterday, or are disorganized, or insist on proceeding without gathering the facts.

The *creative* type individual is future-oriented and gathers most information intuitively. These individuals consider a wide range of possibilities in attempting to solve problems. They are most stressed by people who resist change, are mired in rigid rules and regulations, and focus on useless details, encouraging an environment of stagnation.

The *emotional* type is driven fundamentally by relationships with others. These people's guiding force is how they perceive other people will feel about a given action. For them the greatest stressors are isolation, guilt, and the disapproval or criticism of others.

Once you understand your personality type, you can learn to avoid the situations that are most likely to be stressful to you, or learn not to let them upset you greatly. For example, if you are primarily the emotional type, you should avoid situations in which you are unsupported and isolated. Likewise, the creative type should avoid conditions such as working in a hierarchical corporation, where there are likely to be a lot of rules. The logical type would probably be better off working alone or with others of the same type.

Perhaps it doesn't need to be said, but let me say anyway that physicians are every bit as vulnerable to physical damage from stress, anxiety, isolation, lack of support, and depression as anyone else. I'm sure I'm a typical case.

TRUSTING YOUR HEART MORE THAN YOUR EYES

One of the important sources of stress for me is unavoidable because it is a part of what I do for a living. When I am doing a procedure at the hospital, there are elements which are relatively unpredictable and anxiety-provoking. As I prepare to do a complex angioplasty, I ask myself: Will I be able to open the artery? Will the balloon cross the lesion? Will the artery remain open? What if the patient develops a heart attack and has to go into surgery? For me it is impossible not to feel uneasy about such unpredictabilities. I dislike the reality that I can't control everything. At the same time, I feel responsible for everything that happens. Sometimes a patient reacts in a way I can't control. Still I hold myself responsible.

Yet I can't allow these fears to stop me from doing the best job I can do. And I can't allow them to undermine my own health. Once when I was in the cath lab, a patient's blood pressure began to drop rapidly. For a fraction of a second, *I* felt some chest discomfort. "Boy, Bruno," I said to myself, "does it make sense for you to make yourself sick too?" No, I promised myself. That's not going to happen!

I am no different from you. I must accept personal responsibility for my health. Refusing to give myself adequate time to process my work and life experiences caught up with me a couple of years ago, and I had to take my symptoms of gastric distress to a colleague. I was lucky; it was a warning.

It's not right to pinch our lips and shake the finger at ourselves, though. Most of us have been doing the best we can with the information we have. Usually we have good reasons for the things we do; usually we are driven by loving and being loved— being accepted, supported, connected, and safe. In the next pages I'll discuss ways to control unavoidable stress and refrain from letting it make us sick.

STAYING IN CONTROL

Some people say that getting old is unavoidable but growing is optional. The same principle applies to stress. Stress is part of life—it's even good for us in normal amounts. The problem comes when our levels of stress become so great that we can't handle them, or our coping mechanisms are so poor that even normal levels of stress are overwhelming.

Luckily our bodies give us warning signs when we leave this comfort zone of adaptation to stress. According to Robert Eliot, the body signs can be behavioral, emotional, or physical. There are behavioral patterns that should be signals to you. One is avoidance: isolating yourself; avoiding responsibility and work; using drugs or alcohol excessively; neglecting yourself; and being prone to accidents. Some experience self-destructive behavior in shoplifting, driving carelessly, or instigating relationship problems. Emotional signals include fatigue, anxiety, anger, apathy, irritability, or impatience. The physical signs manifest as muscular tics, muscle tension, cold or sweaty hands, digestive problems, or frequent illness. If we ignore these warning symptoms, the stress will continue to pile up, leaving us open to disease.

Because we are individuals, we each have our special reactions to stress. Some people are lucky; they are born stress hardy. What makes people stress hardy? In part it is their attitude toward the challenges of life. They tend to look at change as a challenge rather than a danger. The stress hardy have a good sense of control and at the same time are able to give up control when necessary. They are committed and have a purpose in life. They tend to be optimistic.

An exceptional heart patient named Marc comes to mind when I think of these qualities. After suffering chest pains he had undergone angioplasty in 1986 and 1988 (in different arteries). Marc told me that he likes to play racquetball three times a week but that recently his doctor had told him that a monitoring test had revealed silent ischemia and was recommending further angioplasty.

Marc, however, calmly refused. He pointed out that he could play ball without problems. Obviously, his doctor's warnings didn't upset him at all. "If I drop dead," he told me, "I will drop dead with a smile on my face on a racquetball court."

Marc also teaches piano daily. He often plays racquetball with younger people, but when he feels tired he lets the other guy win. Instead of allowing the stresses of life to get to him, Marc relaxes and takes care of himself. His cholesterol count is 150, he can walk two or three miles without symptoms, and he recently reduced his weight from 200 to 160 pounds. His hair is black; he has a beautiful smile; his body is well conditioned; and he has a youthful, energetic gait. When his regular physician urged him to start playing racquetball with people his own age, Marc replied, "I can't find them. They are mostly in the cemetery." Marc is eighty-one years old.

How can you learn, like Marc, to become stress hardy? The first step is just realizing that stress is a problem that's possible to handle. Here's one way to look at the stress in your life. Imagine that you have a flame inside you, and that you have a mechanism that governs the intensity of the fire. Handling stress is like adjusting that flame. You can overreact to some situations and be terribly stressed—like turning the flame all the way up to high—or you can react calmly, even to an emergency—remaining cool inside by keeping the flame turned way down.

One way to learn to regulate that internal thermostat is to gain a greater sense of control over your life by becoming more assertive. Assertiveness is the ability to affirm yourself, to state your beliefs, your wants, and your needs. It is the ability to validate yourself in your feelings and thoughts. When you fail to assert yourself, you are giving up the right to live your own life, to pull your own strings. The moment this happens it is easy for stress to get the upper hand.

I am not saying that you should become overbearing or aggressive, only that you need to become conscious of your own rights and be able to state them rationally. You need to worry less about pleasing other people and more about pleasing yourself. For many years I wasn't assertive because I feared displeasing others, and I believe that heart patients often suffer the same problem. Because they are sick, because they are under the care of experts, they don't have the courage to say no to their doctors and yes to themselves.

WHAT YOU DON'T KNOW MAY HURT YOU

I firmly believe that cardiac patients must take the initiative and become as knowledgeable as possible about their conditions and the value of the tests they take. You should know, for instance, that a resting cardiogram may be normal even in someone who has coronary artery disease and that the treadmill test is more meaningful. You should be informed that the thallium stress test is even more accurate, and that the angiogram is the most meaningful of all.

You should be aware that in some small hospitals there are no facilities for angiography, which means that you can't get the tests you need, and this can jeopardize your well-being if you develop complications. So your responsibility includes educating yourself and becoming familiar with the hospitals where you live. It might not be a bad idea to visit your area hospitals and see how you feel about each one. When you go, pay close attention to the quality of the rooms, how the personnel interact with patients, and the strength of the surgical program. You might not want to go so far in checking out your hospital options, but it is essential for you to be aware of the fact that *you have the power to choose*. Exercising this power is assertiveness. In short: Be responsible.

To become more assertive, you must first become aware of the areas in which you do and don't take control of your own destiny. We all have areas where we are confident enough and other areas where our assertiveness could be improved. Some people are more assertive at work and less at home or vice versa. Jack, a patient who had insomnia and appeared extremely stressed out, was able to identify his lack of assertiveness at home as the main source of his stress. "When I go to work, I'm happy," he told me. "I go to the office, it's a different environment. Nobody argues with me. I use the phone, if somebody gives me an argument, I hang up. You know what I'm saying? I can shut them off. But I can't shut my wife off. I can't shut my kid off."

SAY YES! TO YOURSELF

To identify the areas where you have more control, become more aware of your daily behaviors. For instance, how often in a conversation do you refrain from expressing your judgment or ideas? Do you actively participate in discussions, or do you sit back and let others talk? How often do you give ambivalent answers and opinions rather than state exactly where you stand, for fear of being judged or criticized? Whenever you notice yourself behaving in a nonassertive manner, deliberately try to change that behavior. Express your opinions; let yourself be heard. This small step will spill over into other areas of your life.

Another way to become more assertive, paradoxically, is to learn to ask for help when you need it. Nobody likes to appear needy. Many of us would rather deny ourselves almost anything than humbly ask for help. Yet the ability to see our own limitations is a virtue.

Finally, being assertive means understanding and asking for your rights. Your first right is to be happy, to live a normal life, and to follow your dreams. You also have the right to say no if a request is unreasonable, and you have the right to say it without experiencing any guilt. You have the right to make mistakes. You have the right to change your mind. You have the right to choose your own friends and activities. You have the right to say what you wish, as long as it isn't harmful to others. You also have the right to remain silent if you prefer to do so. Most of all, you have the right to be yourself.

I remember Rob, a patient who had a heart attack and then, a few days later, a stroke caused by a blood clot that went from his heart to his brain. As a result, he lost the power of speech, and his once very full life changed overnight to one that seemed marginal. This experience would have destroyed many men, and I was concerned about what would happen to Rob's self-esteem. I needn't have worried. Rob had always had a very strong sense of himself, and he came into my office a few months later with a portable computer. He carried on his side of the conversation by typing words onto the keyboard so I could read them on the screen. He seemed happy, and at the end of our visit he pulled out a picture of a boat he had just bought. When I expressed my astonishment, Rob winked at me and typed out the words "Why not?"

Why not, indeed? Why not be an exceptional heart patient, by being as fully alive, as fully yourself, as Rob is?

HEARTSKILL 6: RELEASING STRESS

The antidote to stress is relaxation. Deep relaxation produces the following effects on your body: Your heart rate and blood pressure drop; your breathing rate and oxygen consumption decline; your brain waves move from the alert beta rhythm to a relaxed alpha rhythm; blood flow to your muscles decreases; more blood is sent to the brain and skin; and a feeling of relaxed warmth and rested alertness spreads through you. *All of these are opposites of the body's responses to stress.*

Later on I will give you several practices for reducing the stress in your life over the long term. But here are four proven ways to stop stress in its tracks. Use any or all of them when you are feeling stressed out.

1. Just concentrate. Research shows that *any* activity that totally absorbs your attention produces the relaxation response in your body. If sitting in a chair with your eyes closed doesn't seem to relax you, or if you just need to get away from worries for a while, schedule an activity that makes you lose track of time and captures your attention in a positive way. Choose knitting, crossword puzzles, gardening—anything that takes you out of yourself and helps you to forget about whatever is worrying you at the moment.

2. Shout "*No!*" Tom Ferguson, physician and author of *The No-Nag, No-Guilt, Do-It-Your-Own-Way Guide to Quitting Smoking*, and psychologist Dennis Waitley, author of *The Psychology of Winning*, suggest using the following technique when the cause of your stress is other people making too many demands on your time and energy. Find a place where you can be by yourself and shout "*No!*" as loudly as you can, or shout it

inside your head. This technique also works for chasing away undesirable or self-defeating thoughts. You may feel silly at first, but you will see it works. With some practice it will become automatic, and you will have laid claim to that high ground which is the envy of both goal and spiritual achievers—thought control.

3. Breathe! Joan Borysenko advises that "if the mind is stormy . . . restoring regular breathing automatically restores our peace of mind." To restore normal breathing, take ten full, slow breaths from the belly. This will bring increased oxygen to your brain and with it a renewed sense of alertness. In addition, deliberate control of breathing forces everything in the body, including the mind, to assume the same controlled, relaxed state.

4. Let the sun in. Sit in a comfortable chair facing the sun through an unshaded window. Close your eyes and, for five minutes or so, simply be aware of the sun shining on your body. Sense the warmth of the sun as the love of God healing you. Let that gentle warmth dissolve any problems within you, and enjoy your togetherness with the infinite power within you.

Chapter Nine

YOUR FAITH AND
YOUR HEART

The soul of God is poured into the world through the thoughts of man.
—Ralph Waldo Emerson

Three hundred years of scientific progress have separated us from the natural connection between healing and the spirit. Yet at one time all healing was the province of religion, and we can still see remnants of this tradition in the details of professional medical dress, treatments and their paraphernalia, places of healing, and the aura surrounding them.

In primitive times all sickness was believed to originate in the supernatural realm. Those who had power over the spirits—the witch doctors—were called upon to deal with illness. These healers used religious artifacts in their healing ceremonies. It was only with the Greek and Roman civilizations that healing became separate from religion. Hippocrates, the revered father of modern medicine, was the first to base medical practice on the principles of inductive philosophy and the natural history of disease. He proved that many diseases could be treated by natural means alone. By the time the Roman Empire declined, the priest-physician had become the secular physician, who followed the Greek tradition of receiving fees for medical attention.

In the Middle Ages most doctors were, again, religious men who accepted without question the teachings of their church. Because belief in demons was a part of Church doctrine, it revitalized the notion that disease is supernatural in origin. Relics and religious paraphernalia again became major instruments of healing.

With the coming of the Scientific Revolution, however, medicine and religion split once and for all. Unfortunately, this separation, according to Manly Hall, author of *Healing: The Divine Art*, has deprived humanity of "a spiritual consolation essential to its well-being."

As we grew more modern, medicine was further removed from the spiritual realm. It is only in very recent years that spiritual elements have once again found their place in medicine, that healing is once again becoming the province of the soul as well as the body.

The truth is that physical health is related to spiritual and emotional health. With all of the emphasis today on physical fitness, we are in danger of becoming physically fit but spiritually unfit. As I've said in previous chapters, there is a growing body of evidence that the inner power of healing is as real and concrete as hypodermic needles and CAT scans. But there are as yet few studies in the field directly addressing spirituality. This is because physicians, like most scientists, shy away from what are called soft data. Soft data are anything outside the realm of physics, mathematics, and so on—the exact sciences. But I firmly believe that no matter how "spirit" is defined—whether in traditional religious terms or as a component of mind—it is necessary to become spiritual in order to become healthy.

In one of the few studies on the subject, a ten-month experiment with 393 coronary patients at San Francisco General Hospital proved that the group who received outside prayer in addition to standard medical treatment did far better than those who received medical treatment alone. Those in the experimental group—who did not know that prayers were being said on their behalf—suffered fewer problems with congestive heart failure, pneumonia, and cardiac arrests, and had a significantly lower mortality rate.

It is difficult to explain such results in conventional scientific terms, but the results are real. As one of my exceptional heart patients, a psychiatrist, put it, "There is an unknown in terms of the intellect: That unknown has sometimes been called God. If you try to analyze it rationally, you get nowhere. I've gone through the proofs of St. Augustine as well as St. Thomas Aquinas, but they don't really hold up; they are not able to prove anything to you. On the other hand, as you go through them, you develop an intuitive grasp of the totality of existence, which becomes an internal conviction without intellectual involvement. Once you come to that, you no longer need any proof, you no longer need explanations, you just know what spirituality means and where you're headed with it."

SPIRITUALITY VERSUS RELIGION

It is very important in any discussion of spirituality to separate the spiritual from the religious. The spiritual is, in my view, a crucial component of every phase of a person's life, while the religious is optional.

So what do I mean by *spiritual*? It seems obvious to me that each of us is much more than just a mind and body hanging together in the same space, like a couple in common-law marriage. Indeed, the mind, body, and spirit are intimately connected and interdependent. To speak of one without considering the others makes no sense. The spiritual, then, in humans (and all living things) is the part we can't see; it energizes the part we can see. We get our word *spirit*, in fact, from the Latin word *spiritus*, meaning "breath," or "life principle." Many people call it the *soul*, a word that comes from the German, meaning the "vital or essential part."

This is the part of ourselves I'm talking about when I refer to spiritual and spirituality: the part that moves me further out into life or pulls me back from it, that feels and has ideas and acts on them, thinking and willing and choosing. Or, to look at it another way, it is the same power and intelligence within me that engineered my physical systems cell by cell and today heals my cuts and grows my hair and fingernails.

You can see that, in the way I'm using it, the word *spiritual* means something more basic than religion. It is the organic bedrock out of which religions are carved. The spiritual *is*. Religions explain, describe, harness, and elaborate on the spiritual. Religion is a pathway to the spiritual domain, but spirituality goes further than religion.

How does spirit tie in with belief? Belief, or appraisal, is considered by some writers, including Joan Borysenko, to be the major factor in the mind-body connection. How I appraise conditions, situations, and circumstances determines what my body does and therefore also determines the quality of my physical well-being. The clinical studies cited at the beginning of Chapter 5 give scientific credence to this notion. Appraisals and the emotions and behaviors they engender produce physiological responses in the neural, endocrine, and immune systems, thus preparing the seedbed for illness or health.

You may think that I'm playing with words here. In previous chapters we've looked at the studies linking state of health with emotions. To me belief, appraisal, meaning—whatever you wish to call it—boils down to the same thing biologically. It is a mental/emotional stand taken by the person that

directs action within the physical self. If the belief/appraisal/
meaning is positive, then the action in the body will also be
positive.

I see this phenomenon over and over in my practice. I know
from my patients that meaning keeps them alive and also draws
them into activities which help them develop as people. The
bottom line is that you must believe there is something to live
for in order to continue to live. For Joan, a seamstress, a severe
heart attack in her late sixties was one more setback in a life of
tragedy. In one eighteen-month period, she lost her daughter,
her mother, and her father. And now she was disabled by heart
disease. Such a tragedy would have embittered many people,
but it only strengthened Joan's faith and sense of purpose. "I've
always prayed," this exceptional heart patient told me. "After
tragedies I prayed that God would help me to be kind and to
understand people."

A widow for several years, Joan keeps busy, finding meaning
in her faith and her friends. "I know people who are so interested in themselves that they can't see anything else," she says.
"They can't reach out and enjoy what they have. That's so sad to
me. I'm sixty-seven, and I know that I can't change the world,
but I can live the best I know how. I have lots of friends who call
me, and I work at church. I have a bridge club. I even have two
boyfriends. I have a lot of faith. I really enjoy life."

FAITH AND HEART DISEASE

As I discussed before, people with healing personalities take care
of their bodies. How simple this sounds! Yet what, exactly, does
it mean in practical terms? The obvious things are diet, exercise,
and giving up smoking. But what other nonscientific means are
there? What about those who rely on prayer, meditation, affirmations, and visualizations? For many patients these, too, are a

way of taking care of the body. Sometimes they are the most important measures of all.

When you are told that you have a heart problem, there is a physical wound and a spiritual wound. As a doctor I can take care of the physical wound. As a teacher I can only help lead you to where you can begin to heal your spiritual wound. Paradoxically, though, I believe that the healing of your physical heart can't take place without the healing of your spiritual heart. The way I see it, clearing the channels of spirituality is equivalent to opening the heart's arteries.

Just as doing physical exercise on a regular basis increases our strength, by doing spiritual practice we develop a sort of spiritual muscle. Bit by bit we gain easier access to the spiritual domain. At the same time our spiritual resources will grow, and eventually we will see that problems are really opportunities to meet God.

FINDING A SPIRITUAL PATH

"Everybody looks for a cataclysmic event like St. Paul being thrown from the horse, or going out and having a vision and being transformed by it. Everybody is looking for that mystical experience that is going to transform their life. It doesn't exist. Forget about it, don't look for it. It occurs rarely. Usually, even when it occurs, you can only attain it if you've prepared yourself appropriately for it."

The speaker here is Sam, a fifty-three-year-old doctor who was a self-described atheist until his heart attack. After he recovered he realized that "there has to be more to all of this and that I had to reevaluate things." Without knowing it, Sam had taken the first steps toward becoming spiritual.

The truth is that you can't *not* be spiritual, because we are spiritual beings whether you choose to believe it or not. Whatever you want to call the spiritual part—your soul, God, or whatever—it is a part of you and becomes an integral aspect of the healing process.

But how do you find God or the infinite? As Sam advises, you must prepare yourself appropriately. You must be aware of the possibilities of the spirit. You can find God by realizing that everything in nature reveals the creator.

In my own case, becoming spiritual was part of a long journey. I have to admit that I was taught as a child to pay attention to my conscience. But I was also supposed to make my conscience match somebody else's rules. I wasn't trained to pay attention to what my spirit wanted, how it felt, and what it needed.

My attunement to my spirit has become an art and a necessity for learning, through trial and error. I've tried many paths, and from each one I have grown a little more spiritual. I began my journey when the practice of medicine, the life dedicated to waiting in a hospital to save the next heart victim, was no longer fulfilling. This happened when I began to realize that what people most needed was not to be healed but to not become sick in the first place. At that time I began to look for my own ultimate meaning and means to contribute to the lives of others.

Dropping the Mask

My search began with spiritual teachers, most notably Carleton Whitehead, Bernie Siegel, and Gerald Jampolsky. From Whitehead I learned to make the connections I needed between thought, feeling, physicality, and spirituality. He then inspired me to think deeply about the healing power of nature and the presence of an intelligence within the body. From Bernie Siegel, who holds support groups for cancer patients, I learned to learn about life, death, and love from my own patients. At the Center for Attitudinal Healing in Tiburon, California, I met Gerald

Jampolsky's patients, terminally ill children who are learning to recover or to die in peace. I was deeply moved by the wisdom of the children and inspired by Jampolsky, who had developed his own spirituality and found a practical way to express his love for others.

In addition to studying with these wise and compassionate teachers, I learned from Science of Mind and Werner Erhard's Forum. From Science of Mind, which is the study of spiritual psychology, I learned that the way you think creates your experience in the world. I learned that my spirituality had been dormant for many, many years and now was seeking expression. And from Werner Erhard's Forum, I began to understand myself far better. I discovered that all my life I have felt that I am not good enough and have overcompensated with my cardiologist act. Once I understood this I felt enormously freed—to be my true self, with myself and with my patients.

When I began to do spiritual work, I found that my spirit expresses its pleasures or its pain in every area of my life. Pleasure tells me when I am already on the right track, following a direction that is productive and good for me, and my health. Pain tells me when something is not working, and also suggests direction by negative assertion—"That feels awful! Stop doing that!"

It is as if there are two realities, the everyday one and the more sublime one. Our spirits live in both realities, but we are most likely to become aware of the spirit in the sublime reality.

Finding a Heart and Yourself

I'm going to tell you a very strange story now that is absolutely true. I had a chance to interview an exceptional heart patient I will call Anna. You may have read about her in a popular magazine or seen her story on television. Anna had been sick with heart and lung disease for many years and had undergone a heart and lung transplant, in which she received the organs of an eighteen-year-old man who had been killed in a motorcycle accident. "It wasn't like what the doctors say, that you just exchange parts and then you are like you were before," she told me. "No way is it like that." She explained that she had been working on a book about her experience, then went on. "It is so strange that I am telling you now, because two days ago, after the culmination of two years of work and preparation of this book, I met with my donor family. It was one of the most wonderful days in my entire life. The authorities would not give me the name of the donor. How I found out was so incredible—he came to me in a dream. He told me his name. He said he was leading me to the light of health. Months later, when I was going down the wrong path, I read his name in an obituary in a newspaper [dating from the time when I had my transplant]. His name was the name I had dreamt. I wrote to his family, and they replied immediately. Then I went over to meet them. It was the family of my heart. It was just miraculous. They took me in and were so hungry to talk to me about him and about me. I am a member of their family now." It may not be scientific, but Anna firmly believes that a part of that young man, the sublime part, still lives within her.

There are many paths to get to that sublime part of oneself. Meditation, visualization, prayer, journaling can all help. There is no one right way for everyone; it will be slightly different for each person. I remember Ezra, a professor of Zen and Eastern philosophy, who found a unique way of combining Eastern philosophy, Western religion, and exercise as part of his regimen to heal his heart. As his wife related it to me, "He was walking on the treadmill at the Y and using a Latin prayer to the Holy Spirit to come dwell in his heart and to heal his heart. But the funny thing was he used it like a mantra, saying it over and over, 'to heal my heart,' while he walked for forty-five minutes. He told me he feels his spirit is growing, and that he feels God is answering his prayers."

When I asked Ezra about his practice, he readily confirmed it and added, "I pray in my own way, not the traditional one. I think it's a deeper prayer than the recitation of the usual prayers, because it's synchronized with my mind and my body being in unity with the world, and the world with the great being out there."

TUNING IN TO THE SUBLIME

Each of these three techniques—affirmation, visualization, and prayer—provides a way to get more in touch with your spiritual self. As you practice each, you are putting your subconscious mind to work. It is like creating a street where you can walk straight and confidently. At the end will be positive results.

Affirmation

Affirmations are, literally, positive statements about ourselves or a situation that we repeat silently or aloud. They provide a way to give a positive energy to what otherwise would be negative thoughts and events. In a very real sense an affirmation is a deliberate way of leading the mind to the state of consciousness you wish to experience. "I always do the best I can" is an example of an affirmation you might create for self-assurance in a work situation that feels stressful. "All is well with me and my affairs" is another.

When repeated regularly, affirmations not only block thoughts you don't want to have but change your thinking in the moment from thoughts that hurt you to thoughts that support you.

You do not need to be religious to use affirmations, but you do need to be open-minded and faithful, because if you think that you don't really deserve the good things you repeat in the affirmations they won't work. If, on the other hand, you faithfully repeat the affirmations, they will change your experience in the same way that repeated drops of water can eventually perforate rock.

Affirmations can be about anything negative in your life. Examples include "I deserve happiness. I am healthy. I have a healthy heart." Whatever positive statement you choose, repeat it silently to yourself several times a day.

Louise Hay, author of *You Can Heal Your Life*, suggests saying affirmations in front of a mirror and noticing any negative thoughts or feelings that come to mind. Becoming aware of these negative messages is important, because then you can bring them into the light and eliminate them.

Visualization

Related to affirmations are visualizations, which take affirmation one step further. In visualization you visualize the good thing that you want as an actuality, existing in the present. This works because your brain experiences the visualization as if it were true. This will help to bring it into your experience.

One of the best uses of visualization is to attain deep relaxation. To practice this visualization, find a quiet place, relax, and close your eyes. Then imagine a beautiful setting where you feel safe and comfortable. Try to imagine the sounds, feelings, smells, and vivid colors. For instance, you might see yourself in the mountains admiring a magnificent view, feeling the air crisp and pure against your skin. Or you might imagine yourself in the summertime under a tree you love, your hair stirred by a gentle breeze. Perhaps you see yourself at the beach, stretched out on the sand, water murmuring just beyond your toes and the sun warming your face. As you place yourself fully in the scene, see yourself relaxing. See yourself happy and at peace.

Prayer

Prayer, whether the traditional verses you learned in childhood or a wordless reaching out to the infinite, is a timeless moment in consciousness. To pray is to be attuned to the consciousness of God within. I find it is easier to pray after relaxation or meditation, when my mind has become still and my creative consciousness is at rest.

I cannot tell you how to pray any more than I can tell you what to believe, but if you have a feeling for the spirit within you and surrounding you, reach out in communion to that spirit with words or feelings. When I pray I feel I can raise my consciousness and see the world and myself from the highest point of view. When I pray I can contemplate the spiritual garden of my mind and see what spiritual values I am cultivating.

Praying is an enriching experience. It is the realization that perfect happiness is already within us and that peace lies in communion with the infinite, not in possession of material goods or worldly success. Prayer makes us more aware that our essence is spiritual and that as spirit we are perfect and ageless. When I have prayed with a patient and we open our eyes and look at each other, we experience a sense of connectedness.

I believe that we have spiritual hearts and that they are never sick. The spiritual heart is a perfect heart, a divine heart. It will live forever. Your spiritual heart has a healing power beyond your understanding. It is a source of the greatest energy, creativity, and love. Show your heart gratitude and take good care of it. Feed it with spiritual thoughts, with moments of friendship, with moments of thanksgiving for being the source of your life.

You need never feel lonely again. Pray with your spiritual heart. Ask God to guide you, to inspire you, to give you the strength to fulfill your creativity and the perseverance you need to continue. Pray for your heart to be filled with the values of friendship, love, and peace.

HEARTSKILL 7: LEARNING TO MEDITATE

Meditation is an ancient technique used to quiet the mind, to allow us to get in touch with our own inner wisdom. In order to achieve this state, it's necessary to focus your attention on the innermost part of yourself. Within this space resides the voice that is always waiting to shed light on your life. It's a small voice, a small light, but so powerful that it can shine into the universe. I believe that this light is an expression of the universal intelligence, that it is part of the Spirit of God.

But whether or not you believe in God, meditation will work for you. Spiritually it will help you to center and become more attuned to yourself. At the physical level it can improve your health in many respects. When you meditate your blood pressure goes down, your pulse and breathing slow, and the oxygen consumption of your whole body decreases. Subjectively you gain a sense of peace, of mental clarity, of control. Meditation increases the production of slow alpha brain waves, causing patterns that are different from states of simple relaxation or sleep.

The benefits of meditation continue beyond the time you do it, so the sense of calmness and control it brings extends through the day. You gain the capacity to choose what to think. You become, in a sense, an observer of yourself and your life. You are no longer overwhelmed by your emotions but able to see them clearly, almost at a distance. To me meditation is like sitting at the edge of a lake where the waters are gently moved by a wind;

gradually the wind falls and I am able to see to the bottom of the lake. All of a sudden, things become clear in my mind.

For meditation to be most beneficial, it must be performed on a regular basis. When you choose to practice is up to you, but I recommend at least once a day, preferably twice, for fifteen to twenty minutes each time. Ideal times to meditate are before breakfast and before dinner. Just find a place and time where you can be alone and undisturbed by the phone or anything else.

Dr. Herbert Benson, Harvard cardiologist and author of *The Relaxation Response*, offers the following technique: Find yourself a comfortable chair and sit with your body relaxed, your hands in your lap, and your eyes closed. The reason for closing your eyes is that 75 percent of all sensations are visual, so just closing your eyes helps the mind to rest. Assume a passive attitude toward your thoughts. That means that if a thought comes into your mind, simply let it go. Don't dwell on it, don't fight it, simply observe it and let it go away.

Next, focus on your breathing: As you breath in and out, concentrate on the feeling of the air going through your nostrils. Focusing on that sensation can help you to eliminate distracting thoughts. Dr. Benson recommends repeating silently to yourself a word each time you breathe out. It can be *God*, *peace*, *love*, or any word that has meaning for you. If you can't think of a specific word, simply use the word *one*. But remember to repeat the word with each breath.

As you practice, keep in mind that it's not important how well you do the meditation. The important part is how consistently you work on it.

If you don't have time to do a full meditation, or if you are especially stressed, you can try what I call a minimeditation. Simply sit in a relaxed position with your eyes closed and follow the procedures I've just described for a few minutes.

Chapter Ten

BODY AND SOUL

Your body is the heart of your soul.
—Kahlil Gibran

When you are learning to be an exceptional heart patient, the body is both the easiest and the most difficult part to take care of. It's the easiest because many problems with the body are obvious. For example, you may be extremely overweight, or so out of shape that you can't even run for a bus. But it's also difficult. One aspect that makes it hard is that many of us wait until our bodies are in terrible shape before taking action. It's also difficult because "taking care of your body" in this youth-oriented culture seems beyond the reach of many of us, requiring hours of exercise and spartanlike dieting.

Well, I'm not going to suggest that you become a marathon runner or start eating only bean sprouts and yogurt. Instead, I'm going to give you some simple guidelines for taking better care of your body and show you how some of my exceptional heart patients do it. Then, in the next chapter I'll explain how to put together your own personalized daily practice, combining regimens for your body, mind, and soul that will help to heal your heart and make you as healthy as possible.

FIVE KEYS FOR HEALTHY LIVING

Here are the five keys I use for myself and my patients to ensure that our bodies are as healthy as possible.

1. Respect your body.
2. Take good care of your body.
3. Keep your body moving.
4. Feed your body healthy food.
5. Drop unnecessary crutches.

As you can see, these are simple precepts—and simpler to follow than you might think. For explanations and guidelines for each of the five keys, read on.

1. Respect your body.

I mean this literally: Respect your body. I told you earlier in this book that your heart talks to you; it tells you what is wrong. The same is true of your whole body. Remember that careful listening is the mark of respect. It's true that the body doesn't use words, but it does have a language of physical signals. Learn that language and pay attention to it. If you find yourself exhausted at the end of the day, for example, this is a message from your body that you are overdoing and need to rest. A stiff neck, lower back pain, all the little signs that we usually ignore, are actually messages from our bodies that all is not well.

Many people, including myself, believe that the body is the temple of God. Whether you believe that or not, you know it is the only body you will ever have. When you look at it that way, it shouldn't be difficult to make your body one of your first priorities.

2. Take good care of your body.

Taking good care of your body is different from the first key, because the first is an attitude, while this one has to do with actions you can take for the good of your body. When I say take good care of your body, I mean at least give it the same quality of care you give your automobile or any other material thing you value. Now it's true that you can't take your body in for an oil change and tune-up. But your body does need a similar, regular evaluation.

First, have a complete physical checkup—weight, blood pressure, and examination of vital organs (heart, lungs, liver, kidneys). Have your doctor give you a blood test that will answer questions such as, What is my cholesterol level? My blood sugar? What is the ratio of HDL to LDL cholesterol? Such numbers are much more important to know than your social security or driver's license numbers. Have your doctor include an electrocardiogram and treadmill test as a part of the checkup. These can give you an indication of when and how much you need to exercise and which forms of exercise are right for you.

Find out as much as you can about the condition of your entire body. How are your eyes, your hearing, your skeletal system, your mouth and teeth? Is your circulation normal? There are practical reasons for learning all these things about yourself: Not only will they tell you where you stand in terms of general health, but they can also dissipate any fear of the so-called silent killers, such as high blood pressure.

Suppose you follow my advice and you receive an indication of an illness that needs immediate attention, such as diabetes. Of course you will follow your doctor's orders. But go beyond that; read all the information you can get your hands on, and also watch any videotapes your physician or organizations such as the American Diabetes Association can provide. I keep a video library at my office, which my patients have told me they deeply appreciate. Being well informed marshals your energies for recovery not only by dissipating fear but by laying before you the wide variety of weapons available for fighting the disease.

3. Keep your body moving.

Live in action. Remember that your body is designed for activity, life, motion. Don't be a couch potato. That only paralyzes both your body and your mind. Remember, too, that the less active you are, the less active you'll be able to be. This is a simple physiological fact.

Why should you be active in the first place? Well, look at it this way. Your heart is a muscle. It is not a jewel that must be kept in a safe deposit box. The more you exercise, the better you will feel. As you feel better, you will behave better and like yourself better. In other words, your feelings will motivate you to improve the quality of your life. You will become more relaxed, less tense, and be able to get rid of stress more easily. You will feel more energetic.

As if that weren't enough, regular exercise is tremendously good for your whole body. Exercise lowers cholesterol. It helps you lose weight, burn calories, and increase metabolism, causing you to consume more calories all day long. If you combine exercise with a moderate calorie-reduced diet, you will lose weight even faster. Exercise helps you relax and sleep better. It's also very beneficial for your heart. In fact, it's so important that the American Heart Association recently upgraded sedentary lifestyle to one of the major risk factors for heart disease. If you are physically inactive, you are 1.9 times more likely to develop heart disease than if you're active, even if all other factors are the same. The well-known cardiologist Dr. Dean Ornish has found that exercise, combined with dietary change and regular stress relief, reduces coronary artery blockage in patients with severe symptoms.

You're probably thinking that you've heard all this before. You may even be thinking, It may be good for me, but I can't possibly find the time to exercise. Besides, I've always hated exercising. Or how about these excuses? Exercise makes me tired. I'm too old to exercise. I've never been good at sports.

It's easy to make up excuses—I know, I do it too. One of my own excuses is that it takes too much time to exercise. But the truth is that exercising gives you *more* time in the long run, because it improves your stamina and helps you sleep better. Besides, you can always work in more activity, whether or not you do formal exercise. If you really don't have time for a workout, then simply avoid elevators. Use the stairs, starting by climbing one floor at a time. Later on I'll give you more suggestions for working exercise into your daily life.

What about the other excuses? Exercise will not make you tired unless you overdo it. Any regular exercise will actually make you more energetic in the long run. You're never too old to exercise. As for not being good at sports, you don't need to practice a sport. In fact, I advise you to choose only exercises that you *enjoy*. Jogging, for example, is said to add years to your life—but I have heard that those extra years are usually spent jogging! Far better for me at least is walking early in the day at my own pace. If the exercise you choose is just a prescription the doctor told you to practice every morning at six, it won't work, because you won't stay with it.

If you really hate all kinds of formal exercise (or believe you do—you may come to change your mind), try the stretching approach of such Eastern traditions as yoga or tai chi. These slow, controlled movements not only maintain muscle and joint health but evoke a natural meditative relaxation for most people.

You say you still don't like to exercise? Maybe you don't know how many choices there are. You can walk, jog, swim, golf, bowl, dance, do Jazzercise, play tennis, play softball, garden. Whatever you choose, the most important factor is to get moving. I've told you that my exceptional heart patients all have found their own ways to a better life, but I do have to say that nearly all of them include at least some form of exercise. One patient who relies on exercise especially is Mr. Walton, who at age seventy-six is as active as a man half his age. He had experienced chest pain, and tests revealed that he'd suffered a heart attack. When doctors wanted to put him in the hospital, he refused. "I don't believe it," he told me flatly.

Every day he gets some form of exercise. "I work out, I swim, lift weights, play a little basketball," he says. "Some days I just take a fast walk in the street for forty-five minutes or so. It's not at all hard. I listen to my body. If my body feels like stopping, I stop. If it doesn't, I keep on going."

When I asked Mr. Walton what kept him going, how he made himself continue to be so active, he emphasized, "Most people my age just fall asleep. I go to the club, I see them playing cards, it makes me want to go work out. I don't want to be like them."

I pointed out that in today's busy world not everyone has time to work out. Mr. Walton practically exploded. "If you can find time to work and time to eat," he demanded, "why can't you find time to exercise? If you're going to work eight hours a day, why can't you find one or two hours to work out?"

GETTING STARTED. The very first thing you should do before beginning an exercise program is to seek a cardiologist or physician and have a checkup to assess your heart's present health.

So now you're ready to start your new exercise program. You may have many more questions, especially if you've never exercised regularly before. For example, what should you wear? My suggestion is loose, comfortable clothing. Avoid rubber or plastic workout suits, which can cause you to become overheated. One good rule is that if working out in cold weather, you should wear one layer less than you would ordinarily wear outdoors. If the day is hot and humid, it's better to exercise early in the morning or in the evening, and to drink plenty of water.

As for how long to exercise, that will vary from person to person. Whatever you do, and however long you choose to do it, remember to start with a warmup period, let's say five minutes, and then a cooldown period, also five minutes. In between, exercise for seven to ten minutes or whatever your energy level permits. Your ultimate goal should be to work up to a total time—including warmup, cooldown, and exercise—of thirty to sixty minutes, three times a week. But remember that any amount of exercise is better than none. Also bear in mind that getting in condition is a gradual process. It has probably taken you many years to get out of shape, so you can't expect to get in good condition in a week or two.

How hard should you exercise? The best idea is to exercise at your target heart rate, or between 50 and 75 percent of your maximum heart rate. Guidelines for taking your pulse and estimating your target heart rate are in Chapter 1. Just as an example, if you are sixty, your heart should beat during exercise at between 80 and 120 beats per minute. But you don't really need to worry about those numbers. A practical guideline is to work hard enough so that you breathe faster and break out in a sweat, but not so hard that you can't talk while exercising.

If you experience any symptoms while you are exercising, such as light-headedness or chest discomfort or irregular heartbeat, stop immediately and consult your doctor as soon as possible.

CHOOSING YOUR EXERCISE. There are many types of exercises. Most can be divided into three categories, each of which has different effects on the body.

Aerobic exercise. Aerobic exercise is perhaps the most important sort of exercise for cardiac patients because it can condition your heart better than other exercises. Aerobic exercises specifically involve your heart, lungs, and circulatory system by causing you to work the big muscles of your body and breathe deeply. These exercises include jogging, walking, swimming, bicycling, stationary bicycling, and using the treadmill, as well as aerobic dancing and low-impact aerobics classes. There are many good books that will tell you how to get started with an aerobics program. There are also a number of aerobics classes at every gym and Y, and usually you can find aerobics classes especially for heart patients.

Try to do an aerobic exercise three or four times a week for at least fifteen or twenty minutes each time. If you can, work up to half an hour each time. It will make you feel better, clear your head, and relax you while it's conditioning your body. When you're starting, the slower you go the better. This is partly so your body will have a chance to adjust to the increased workload and partly to prevent you from getting burned out. Many people beginning to exercise become too impatient and overdo it; then they have sore muscles and decide exercise isn't for them. Don't make this mistake.

Stretching. The gentle stretches of yoga, tai chi, and other Eastern exercises are good for both the body and the soul. They are different from old-fashioned calisthenic stretches, which involve sudden, sharp, or bouncing movements. Instead they are slow and steady, and each one is held for a while, leading to a meditative state. There are many books and classes available on these exercises.

Yoga in particular is appropriate for heart patients because its focus is both physical and spiritual. Although the techniques demand discipline and faithful practice, the benefits can be immense. Regular practice of yoga improves the balance, strength, and flexibility of the body and promotes discipline and calmness of the mind. Many yoga classes also include breathing exercises, which are quieting and energizing simultaneously.

Whether or not you decide to do formal stretching exercises, it's always a good idea to do a bit of stretching every day, as a warmup before your aerobic exercise and first thing in the morning. It will keep your muscles and joints limber. Just stretch, don't bounce, and hold the stretch until you feel a good pull in your muscles.

Strength training. Strength training includes any exercise that is designed to strengthen your muscles, such as calisthenics, weight lifting, or use of weight-training machines. It is essential that you receive professional strength or weight training instruction before you begin. It's also important to check with a physician before beginning a weight-training regimen because the effort of lifting weights can cause your blood pressure to rise. This is especially true of isometric exercises, which I don't recommend. However, if your doctor gives you an okay, and you enjoy it, weight training can be fun and good for you. It's especially helpful for older women, most of whom have atrophied muscles that can make it impossible to carry or move even lightweight objects. The strength you gain from weight training can help your self-esteem, and there is growing evidence that weight training can help to prevent osteoporosis.

If you decide to do strength training, working out one to three times a week for half an hour is plenty. Be sure to allow a day or more between workouts.

Lifestyle exercises and sports. All sports are good: tennis, golf without a golf cart, badminton, whatever you enjoy. There are many ways to work exercise into your life aside from planned sports as well. I already mentioned taking the stairs rather than the elevator. When you go to work or go shopping, instead of parking right behind the door, park at the end of the parking lot or even a few blocks away. Whenever I go to church I see cars parked just across from the entrance and I have to shake my head. Why would people go to so much trouble to avoid a little exercise? Gardening is also a good way to work physical activity into your life, especially the vigorous activities of raking and mowing with a hand mower.

4. Feed your body healthy food.

Although this may seem obvious, for many people it appears difficult or even unnecessary to feed the body healthy food. After all, if you love well-marbled steaks, you may wonder how your body can do without them. A better question is how your body manages to put up with them. Our adaptable body chemistry can adjust to any ongoing situation, including a diet full of foods that may be destructive. Likewise, adjusting to new, positive eating habits may cause your body to protest for a while, and such changes may merit psychological and social support. That's why I urge that you make any dietary changes under the active supervision of a partner-physician who understands your goals *and* your real difficulties. There are effective support groups and programs for people who love themselves enough to change the way they eat.

The truth is that you really are what you eat. Studies now show that diet can lower blood cholesterol and can greatly reduce further buildup. Clear links have also been found between dietary factors and some forms of mental and emotional illnesses.

You are the one who has to find out what *your* body needs. If you are diabetic, for instance, your body will have different needs than the body of someone who has hypertension, has arteriosclerosis, or is pregnant.

EATING A HEALTHY AND DELICIOUS DIET. A healthy diet for the heart is a low-fat diet for two reasons. First, eating a lot of fatty junk food contributes to excess weight, which is bad for your heart. Second, the same kind of food is known to contribute to the substances that clog arteries. Most of us are well aware of the problem of excess weight—an estimated 47 million American adults are at least 20 percent over their desirable weight. Weighing 30 percent or more above your desirable weight is one of the risk factors for heart disease.

I am convinced that one reason so many people have bad diets is that they don't really pay attention to their food. It's just so easy to go to a fast-food restaurant and order a hamburger, fries, and a thick shake. One of my exceptional heart patients, Ray, had a heart attack at the age of thirty-eight. Before he got sick he always considered himself healthy. "But," he admits, "I realize now I had no one to blame but myself. I was a smoker, and, now that I think about it, my diet was atrocious. I used to live on fast-food hamburgers and tacos, and with my wife working full-time we used to come home and just throw something frozen in the oven or go out for fast food. Now I watch myself, eat more vegetables, and try and stay away from red meat."

Ray has also become more conscious of what everyone in his family eats. "My younger boy is slightly overweight," he told me, "even though he's athletic. When I see him eating a pizza, I tell him he shouldn't eat too much of it, so he won't have the same problems I had when he gets to be forty years old."

Like Ray, you may be surprised to find that it's nearly as easy to eat in a way that's healthy for your heart. All you need to do is follow a few simple guidelines.

First, keep the fat low. The American Heart Association recommends that no more than 30 percent of calories come from
fat. This isn't as hard to achieve as you might think—cut back
on fried foods, red meat, rich dressings for your salads and vegetables. Choose instead from a variety of delicious low-fat
foods, such as fresh fruits and vegetables, poultry and seafood,
and the starchy foods, such as cereals, breads, grains, and
beans. If you eat dairy foods, choose skim milk and other low-
fat products.

Second, go easy on the salt shaker. So many people shake salt
on their food before even tasting it. That can cause elevated
blood pressure in susceptible people. It also keeps you from tasting your food.

Don't use parties or restaurants as an excuse to go back to old,
unhealthy ways of eating. One of my exceptional heart patients,
who is eighty-one, has perfected his technique for sticking to his
healthy diet wherever he is. "When I'm going to a restaurant,"
he told me, "I'll call up the owner first and ask him to cook for
me some special meal, like having the white part of the eggs
with vegetables for an omelet." His blue eyes crinkled and then
he laughed. "Of course not everybody's cooperative; I've had to
walk out of a couple of restaurants. But the ones I've gone to
awhile, they know me now. I walk in, and they have my healthy
meal all ready for me."

Apart from the guidelines I've mentioned, my best advice for
healthy eating is to eat what you like. I believe that the ideal diet
is a mixed one. Many people exaggerate their dietary regimens
and feed themselves as if they were sick. It's true that some of
the stricter dietary regimens seem very healthful, but I don't
remember interviewing any patient who lived a long life—to age
eighty-five or older—who ever told me he or she had followed,
for example, a very strict vegetarian diet. Most of them had a
mixed diet; they ate everything, but in moderation.

5. Drop unnecessary crutches, such as smoking, overeating, and excessive use of alcohol.

Some people call smoking, overeating, and excessive use of alcohol addictions, but I prefer to think of them as crutches because I believe they are unnecessary bad habits that can be changed once we understand them for what they are. H. Milkman, writing in *Psychology Today*, advises that "it is the experience that we are addicted to . . . the specific thing you crave is just the trigger for that experience." What we usually are really craving, he says, is stimulation, relaxation, and/or avoidance of reality.

Too much use of these crutches will create tolerance, so that an ever-larger boost is required to produce the desired experience. In diseases such as alcoholism or drug abuse, the physical craving may become a true addiction, getting progressively demanding and destructive until crippling and finally death result.

Modern medical thinking is finally coming out of the dark ages about such diseases. We know that addiction is not a person's fault but a mismatch of substance and body chemistry that starts a noxious cycle. Generally, the person is trapped in an addiction long before she or he is aware of it; awareness comes only when critical changes become apparent in the body or behavior. Fortunately, such diseases are highly treatable. Alcoholics Anonymous, for example, has proven over the past fifty years that those who really want to get well can.

Even chronic illnesses can become crutches. The patient may come to "need" the illness to justify lack of participation in family life, refusal to work or to live up to his full potential. Likewise, family members can often develop an unconscious need for another's chronic illness. Both the sufferer and the family unwittingly and mutually weave a fabric—made up of guilt, shame, and fear. I have a friend whose mother's alcoholism shielded her, she says, from the difficulties of living an authentic life on her own. She didn't have to worry about closeness with a boyfriend or working harder to advance in her career—how could she? She had to take care of her alcoholic mother. She thus had an investment in her mother remaining an alcoholic.

If you love yourself and your own life enough to challenge your crutch—whatever it is—you will probably have a better chance of success if you discuss your intention with family members first. Preparing them will help them be open to the changes they also will have to make.

Some crutches are less obvious. Most of us have cravings or habits that are not severe enough to cause addictions but are not especially good for us either, if only because they keep us from something better, healthier, and more productive. Examples might be watching TV regardless of what is on or shopping when we don't need anything.

With a little observation, we can locate the experiences triggered by habits and cravings, and find nondestructive ways of meeting those needs. Most cravings, as we've discussed, come from a need for arousal or relaxation, which can be achieved in other ways. For example, many ex-smokers have found that substituting a brisk walk for a cigarette helps reduce their cravings. Likewise, beginning a regular regimen of meditation can confer a calmness that makes withdrawal symptoms from an addiction less distressing.

GIVING UP SMOKING AS A GIFT TO YOURSELF. My experiences with smokers stand out vividly in my mind. I remember as a medical student I went to see my uncle in the hospital. He was a heavy smoker, and both of his legs had to be amputated. I was told that even at that stage he was continuing to smoke, and finally he died of smoke-related illness.

The second patient that comes to mind is one I went to see in the hospital after he had been diagnosed as having cancer of the lungs. Even though he was in the terminal stage of illness, his room was full of smoke. He died in smoke.

The third was a younger man, in his fifties or so, who assured me that he smoked but didn't inhale. His chest X ray showed a mass in his lung, and it was a tumor. Even though he fought, a few months later he died. I remember that when I told him he had a lung tumor, he looked into my eyes and said, "I regret the first time I ever touched a cigarette."

I am looking at a book entitled *Kids Say Don't Smoke*, which contains posters from a smoke-free ad contest. One poster shows Snoopy, sleeping, surrounded by stars and the moon and the words "Dream of a world without cigarettes." Another shows a pack of cigarettes; on each cigarette is a word, such as *fun, relax, mature, popular.* Underneath is written, "Pack of lies."

When even children know how harmful tobacco is, why do so many people still get addicted to it? Part of the reason is the messages of advertising. Part of it is the physiological effect of nicotine. It can give a feeling of calmness and relaxation. But the cost is that each cigarette takes away five to twenty minutes of life. The carbon monoxide in cigarette smoke reduces the oxygen available to your heart; your blood platelets then become sticky, increasing your tendency to form clots. As a consequence of smoking, your arteries become narrower.

If you smoke more than a pack a day, in fact, your risk of heart attack doubles. Switching to low-tar cigarettes or cigarettes with filters is no good. They are even worse, because they have less nicotine, so you're more likely to take deeper breaths and longer puffs. Also, carbon monoxide is not filtered out.

I have seen people who have had a heart attack and still continued to smoke. Since I have never smoked regularly, I don't know what it's like to give the habit up, but I do know that many, many of my patients have done so and have almost immediately started feeling better.

The American Heart Association is one of many organizations

that offer guidelines to help you stop smoking. Here are some of their suggestions.

First, be aware that there are circumstances, called triggers, that evoke a desire to smoke. The most common are watching TV, having a cup of coffee, being under pressure, feeling lonely, finishing a meal, having an argument, driving a car. Although you can't avoid all of these triggers, avoid the ones you can. Especially, for the first few weeks, avoid people who smoke. Beginning an exercise program can be helpful, as can putting something, such as a stick of gum, in your mouth. Also, try some of the relaxation techniques offered in Chapter 8, or even meditate instead of smoking. Use anything you can, including positive thinking or social support for help to break this destructive habit.

Another suggestion is to sign a contract with yourself, promising to stop on such and such a day and then keeping your word. Remember that the promise is not just to you but to your family, your children, and your whole future life. Think of how many more things you can do if you don't smoke; think also of how much money you will save.

Most of my patients quit smoking cold turkey. Many of them quit only after having a heart attack or open-heart surgery. But why wait? Enroll in a stop-smoking class now. These are offered free or for very little money through the Heart Association or at local Y's. Or talk to your doctor about the nicotine patch, which has helped some stop smoking.

Chapter Eleven

PUTTING IT ALL

TOGETHER

Do what you can with what you have where you are.
—Theodore Roosevelt

aily practice consists of the activities that you do every day, or nearly so, to keep your heart healthy or to heal it. This is not a rigid program in which you must do so much of a certain kind of exercise and eat exactly so many calories of a certain food. Rather my exceptional heart patients have taught me that everyone's daily practice is different and that the best thing for your heart is to create your own combination of physical, mental, and spiritual healing exercises. For example, one patient I know combines daily prayer with long walks. Another does meditation and, when she can find the time, likes to play golf and tennis. She is an accomplished cook and has learned how to prepare gourmet-tasting, low-fat meals.

Peter, an exceptional heart patient who had a heart attack at the age of forty-eight, decided to take his own health in hand, and now, six years later, he is symptom free and appears to be in great shape. The other day I asked him about his daily practice, and he told me that he not only does a half-hour gym routine every morning but also follows Dr. Dean Ornish's vegetarian diet, eating skim milk, egg whites, and other low-fat foods. In addition to these healthy physical practices, he meditates from fifteen minutes to a half hour a day and reads inspirational books.

FINDING PEACE IN MY STRESSED HEART

Before I go on and give you the choices for devising your personal plan, let me tell you about my own daily practice. After all, we physicians are always giving prescriptions or advice, but we seldom share very much of ourselves, so I'd like to share this with you.

My practice, when I wake up in the morning—usually about 6:00 or so—is to go to my study and read some inspirational material. Then I sit down and meditate for fifteen or twenty minutes. I have a comfortable chair there, just perfect for this activity, from which I love to look through the little diamond-shaped panes of my windows at the trees, bushes, and wildlife on my front lawn in the early light of a new day.

There are many forms of meditation. I use Dr. Benson's relaxation technique, which is described in full in Chapter 9. Why do I meditate? Because whenever I do I feel better, physically and mentally. The day goes differently. I find more time for myself, things fall into place in the right order, and I have more mental clarity. Meditation costs nothing, and it is immensely more beneficial than medication for the same results. The truth is that we have our own Valium within. All you have to do is sit down, close your eyes, follow the instructions, and find your inner peace.

I have to be honest with you. I don't meditate every day, but I do it as many days as I can, almost always in the morning. And in the evening before dinner, I close my eyes for at least a mini-meditation.

I believe the world would change for the better if everyone

started meditating. I would even recommend it for children. Why not? They have their own stresses, especially teenagers. They often don't know where to turn for answers to their questions, and they can develop severe health problems, such as hypertension, obesity, diabetes, or even heart disease as a result. Thus some of them die prematurely. Beginning meditation at an early age could avert so many bad habits and make people's lives so much better.

The second part of my daily practice consists of exercise. My way of exercising is relatively simple. Nearly every morning I do twenty to twenty-five pushups and about thirty bent-legged situps. I do a little bit of stretching. My whole routine takes only a few minutes.

During the day, in the hospital, I avoid the elevator, and several times I go up and down the six flights of stairs. My weekly exercise is playing tennis early in the morning. I love it, and I'm trying to do it more often. I also like to walk when the weather is good, usually either in the morning or after dinner. There's no special routine or way to walk—I'm not a daily jogger or a marathon runner or any such thing. I used to do that years ago, but I injured myself. So instead I just take a walk with myself. It helps me to be alone, to observe the flowers and my neighbors.

I think it is immensely beneficial to all of us to just be with ourselves for a little bit every day. As I walk I think about what I am doing, how I am developing spiritually, how my plans are going, and sometimes I pray. I express gratitude for what God gives to me, and I ask to be guided. I have even prayed to finish this book soon, because I feel people need it. So you can see that even though I'm talking about physical exercise, in a way this is spiritual too.

There are other activities I do for exercise. I have a stationary bike, and I sometimes ride on it for twenty minutes or so, mostly to get myself into better shape for tennis. In the summer I love to swim, sail, and windsurf. I do all these sports not only because they are good for me but because I love them and they give me vital energy.

My diet is also rather relaxed, although I do watch what I eat. In general, I have a simple breakfast—cereal, sometimes with a banana. For lunch I have soup or something else light, because I have to continue to work after lunch and if I ate heavily I would fall asleep. For dinner I have pasta or some meat, with vegetables and fruit. I have maybe one egg a week. I like to use some olive oil to season my salad, and I love all types of fruits. This sounds very healthy, and I suppose it is, but I have some indulgences too. I have a weakness for espresso, preferably made as cappuccino, and I often have one in the afternoon or after dinner.

I feel comfortable with what I eat and not at all restricted. I enjoy a variety of foods. I have never been crazy about steaks; I prefer chicken or fish. Occasionally I have a small piece of cheese, and I love something sweet for dessert, but not on a regular basis.

My final indulgence is now and then to have half a glass or less of wine with dinner. I prefer white wine, and I believe a little wine with meals is beneficial. It is relaxing, it helps digestion, it raises good cholesterol, and it can improve the mood. As you see, my daily practice is very flexible, suiting my personality and lifestyle. It seems to be working. A few days ago I took a treadmill test: I was able to complete the most difficult protocol, proving that my heart is healthy without my following any sort of rigid program.

PLANNING A DAILY PRACTICE
THAT SUITS YOUR LIFE

You are probably already doing some things that are good for your heart. Maybe you eat a low-fat diet, or maybe you love to get exercise. To plan a daily practice, list the activities you are already doing and then think of areas where you need improvement. For example, you may be deeply spiritual and go to church on a regular basis, but if you are also a couch potato you should try to add some movement to your life. Remember that the catchwords are moderation, variety, and flexibility.

To help you discover the areas where you may need more work, take the following two inventories. The physical inventory will help you assess your physical state and determine the sorts of physical activities that can help your heart. The spiritual inventory will help you discover your strengths and weaknesses in the spiritual area and suggest what you can do to balance that part of your life.

Do you need to lose weight? To exercise more? Unless you feel that your body is in the best shape it could possibly be in, this physical inventory will help you pinpoint the areas where you need to work harder to be as healthy as possible. Answer the following questions, thinking about your answers and the reasons for them.

YOUR PHYSICAL INVENTORY

1. What size pants or skirt do you wear now, and what size did you wear when you were eighteen?

2. What vigorous activities did you do as a teenager, and which ones do you do now? What vigorous activities have you added? (Include all formal exercise as well as sports.)

3. How do you relax? List five things you regularly do to relax your body. (Include choices such as time in a hot tub or napping.)

4. What physical discomforts or complaints do you experience frequently that are not important enough to warrant seeing a doctor?

5. What is your blood pressure? What are your cholesterol and blood sugar counts?

6. When you look at yourself in a mirror, what do you love and what do you want to change? Why?

7. What new kinds of foods and new ways of cooking are you interested in? If you aren't interested in any currently, what ones do you think you could learn to enjoy?

8. What is your idea of a really great dinner? Is there any part that you regret the next day?

9. When was the last time you changed your hairstyle or your way of dressing? How often do you buy something new to wear?

10. In what way would you like to see your health improved by this time next year?

Evaluating Your Physical Inventory

This inventory gives you clues about the things you are now doing that are positive, as well as those that you would benefit by changing. Questions 1 and 2 ask you to compare your physical condition now with your condition when you were younger. Take an honest look at yourself and note the ways your body has changed (fatter, thinner) and how your level of activity today compares with that when you were a teenager.

Question 3 is extremely important. If you cannot list at least five *healthful* things that you regularly do to relax your body, it should be a clear message to you: Begin to add some!

Questions 4 and 5 relate to how well you know your body and understand its health. If you can't come up with the numbers asked for in Question 5, it's time to make an appointment for a general checkup.

Question 6 is related to the first two questions. Again, be honest. Would you look better if you lost some weight? Or are you pleased with how well you have kept yourself in shape?

Questions 7 and 8 explore your eating habits and give you the opportunity to branch out and try new, healthy ways of eating. If you can't even imagine a diet different from the one you have now but suspect your current habits aren't heart healthy, go back and review the diet section in the last chapter.

Questions 9 and 10 both have to do with your self-esteem and the goals you should be setting for a healthier life. Think carefully about the answers to Question 10, and write these new goals down. Remember that naming goals and making them manifest in writing is the first step toward achieving them.

The spiritual inventory contains the key to your future. It will tell you where you connect with meaning and what your appraisal and perception of value in your life are. Deep personal meaning is often difficult to express. In many ways it is taken for granted. Your spiritual inventory will show you where you are already living out of deep personal meaning, in which areas of your life you find it, and perhaps some areas in which you feel a need for more expression of it. It will also guide you toward the practices that can best enable you to further develop your spiritual side.

As I discussed in Chapter 9, meaning is the best way to begin to talk about spirituality. It is from meaning (purpose, goals, values) that your real drive for living comes. The appraisal of meaning is both your spiritual life and its shape. You are spiritually activated by meaning. Seen in that way, natural expressions of spirituality are not that hard to locate; with a little practice the spiritual can be separated from the cultural—meaning given to you by someone else, rather than that which emerges spontaneously from within you.

To find your own core of spirituality, you need to discover what you deeply care about. For me personally, such values include skiing on a bright afternoon, hearing my son Max's school speech, and talking to a group of businessmen about how to protect their hearts. To me these are all spiritual activities because they are all coming from places of deep meaning to me.

To find your own center of spirituality, answer the following questions. As with the other inventories in this book, there are no right or wrong answers. Instead, the questions are designed to guide you. By continuing or beginning activities that relate to the areas where you have your own deepest meaning, you will be able to expand and develop your spiritual side.

If you find that you cannot easily answer any of these questions, I suggest that you try some of the spiritual practices described in Chapter 9: affirmation, visualization, prayer, meditation, whatever you are comfortable with. They will help you become aware of your own deeper self. Or try this exercise, which I often recommend to my heart patients:

To learn to have access to the higher self, close your eyes and go back in memory to one of the moments when you felt especially happy, when you felt that you were really you, when the most genuine, spontaneous, and natural part of yourself was manifested. Reexperience that moment as clearly as you can. Include all the sensory awareness you recall from it. Let yourself be happy again, let yourself be the real you again. When you open your eyes, adjust yourself to the present, recall the exercise you have just done, and think: Isn't it fantastic to know that this real you is still within you?

YOUR SPIRITUAL INVENTORY

1. What people, places, and events make you feel better about yourself and life after you have contact with them?

2. Which activities make you lose track of time?

3. What is it about these people, places, and events that explains their positive effect on you?

4. What five life accomplishments would you like to be able to list to your credit? Why?

5. Do you go to church now? Why?

6. If you went to church when you were small, what did you like about it? From which activities in your life do you get a similar feeling?

7. In what places and during which activities do you feel drawn beyond yourself and connected to others as part of a larger whole?

8. What is happiness? What do you need to have it?

9. List without judgment important aspirations you had in childhood, adolescence, young adulthood, middle age, and now. What qualities do these aspirations represent to you?

10. Which of these desires is represented in your present life? Where and how? Which have not yet appeared?

Evaluating Your Spiritual Inventory

Since this exercise is designed to get you in touch with your deepest values, you can look on your answers as a sort of guide to activities and pursuits that will bring you closer to your true spirituality. For example, Questions 1 and 2 provide you with a list of people, places, and events that are deeply meaningful to you. Spending more time with these people and going to these places and events will enrich your life spiritually as well as socially. When you begin to explore what it is about these experiences that explains their positive effect on you (Question 3), you will gain a key to the values that hold the deepest meaning for you.

Question 4 gives you an opportunity to review the goals that you have already accomplished as well as those you have yet to attain. Be proud of those life goals already achieved and resolve to spend more of your physical and mental energy on the ones you have not yet met. Or you may decide in reviewing your goals that some of them are no longer as important as they once were and that you can let them go.

Questions 5, 6, and 7 give you an opportunity to examine your feelings about formal religion and offer you an opportunity to explore alternative ways to express your spirituality. The answers to Question 7 in particular offer valuable clues to your own spirituality.

The remaining questions should be evaluated in the same way. Each offers you clues to what your spirit, the real you, is seeking in this life. Question 10 gives you a kind of map of where and how those values are now manifesting themselves in your life and invites you to bring more of them into your daily routine.

Chapter Twelve

MY PATIENTS
ALWAYS ASK ME

Don't deny the diagnosis.
Try to defy the verdict.
—Norman Cousins

n this chapter are the answers to the questions my patients ask me most often about heart disease and healthy living habits.

DO WOMEN NEED TO BE CONCERNED ABOUT HEART DISEASE?

The answer to this question, sadly, is a resounding yes. Although heart attack is more common in younger men, statistics show that women's risk begins to climb after menopause and equals that of men by age sixty-five. In fact, heart and blood vessel disease combined are the leading cause of death in women. Each year 250,000 women die of heart disease, more than twice the number who die from all forms of cancer combined. While the average woman has a one in eleven chance of contracting breast cancer, her chances of contracting heart disease are one in two.

As in men, the leading causes of heart disease in women are high cholesterol, high blood pressure, and cigarette smoking. For women, menopause becomes another risk factor, but it's not known for certain if this is because high levels of estrogen have a protective effect. Although younger women, for whatever reason, aren't as likely to develop heart disease as men, once a woman has a heart attack, she is twice as likely to die within the first week as a man of comparable age.

Women also have some different risk factors than men, among them the fact that women smokers who also use oral contraceptives are up to thirty-nine times more likely to have a heart attack. Women have higher triglyceride levels, which predispose them to heart disease. Diabetic women have twice the incidence of coronary disease of other women. Premenopausal diabetic women have the same risk for heart disease as men.

Even women without known risk factors may suffer from extreme stress that can contribute to heart disease. Because they play so many roles in life—mother, worker, caretaker—many women don't take proper care of themselves. When they become ill, they keep working. At the end of the day, when the man of the house often relaxes, his working wife begins her second work shift, in the home. One study found that after 5:00 P.M. men's levels of stress hormones fall dramatically, while women's hormones and blood pressure are elevated. The consequence of all this stress is that many women get less sleep than men, weigh more, have less physical activity, are more Type A, and smoke more.

Why aren't these facts better known? In part, it's because women seldom have a heart attack before menopause, and in part because most studies and publicity on heart disease focus on middle-aged men. Another reason is that women's symptoms are somewhat different from men's. In two-thirds of men, the first symptom of heart disease is likely to be a heart attack or sudden death. In over half of all women, the first symptom is angina, which may be experienced as nausea or vague chest pains and thus may be mistaken for some other ailment. There is also evidence that electrocardiograms and some other tests for diagnosing heart disease are less reliable when used on women, and the number of false positive results is higher for women.

There is some evidence that estrogen replacement therapy may help prevent heart disease in postmenopausal women, but this therapy may promote uterine and breast cancer. In any case, the good news is that women respond every bit as well as men do to changes in lifestyle aimed toward improving the heart's health. If you are a woman concerned about your heart, I suggest you especially apply the advice in this book. Eat and exercise sensibly, learn to relax, give up your crutches, discover your spiritual self.

CAN ASPIRIN REALLY PREVENT HEART ATTACKS?

Aspirin has been proved to reduce blood clots, which can lodge in narrowed arteries and cause heart attacks. But aspirin doesn't do anything about cholesterol.

A study published in *The New England Journal of Medicine* showed that people who take one aspirin every other day can substantially reduce the risk of heart disease. Aspirin appears to be especially effective in preventing a *second* heart attack.

On the negative side, some people are allergic to aspirin, and taking too much aspirin can cause internal bleeding or kidney disease.

MY DOCTOR GIVES ME SO MANY MEDICATIONS. HOW CAN I TELL IF THEY'RE THE RIGHT ONES?

We physicians sometimes tend to give too many medications. If a patient has high blood pressure, for example, I would try to find out why before giving out pills. I would also advise the patient first to reduce salt intake, lose weight if necessary, and start exercise. That will often do the trick. It's my experience that tension, too, plays a role in causing high blood pressure.

The basic problem with overmedication is that medications can interact with one another, reducing the effectiveness of all of them. The best solution is periodically to review with your doctor the medicines you are taking to be sure that all are appropriate for your present condition.

WHAT IS CHOLESTEROL AND WHY IS IT SO IMPORTANT?

Cholesterol is a fatlike substance that is used by every cell in the body to form cell membranes. It is also utilized to create some hormones and other vital bodily chemicals. Cholesterol in the blood transports fats from the liver to the cells for storage. So you can see that it is a vital substance, so important, in fact, that the liver manufactures all the cholesterol we need, about one gram a day.

The problem comes when we take in more cholesterol than we need, and this is unfortunately very easy to do. Cholesterol is found in all animal products, including meat, eggs, fish, poultry, and all dairy products. Foods from plants do not contain cholesterol. So if you see a bag of potato chips with a label saying, "Contains No Cholesterol!" you can laugh; of course potatoes don't contain cholesterol. However, those potato chips do contain high amounts of fat, which can also increase the blood cholesterol level.

You have probably heard about LDL and HDL cholesterol. These refer to the special molecules that transport cholesterol and fats through the blood. Low-density lipoproteins (LDL) carry cholesterol from the liver to the body tissues, while high-density lipoproteins (HDL) carry cholesterol from the arteries to the liver. If you have too many LDLs relative to HDLs, excess cholesterol will tend to be deposited on your arterial walls, leading to arteriosclerosis. The HDL is often known as good cholesterol because it can remove the bad LDL cholesterol from the arterial walls and return it to the liver for excretion. The normal value for blood HDL should be more than 35. The normal value for LDL should be less than 130 and in patients with coronary disease, less than 100.

As for total cholesterol, the risk of heart disease decreases when the cholesterol level is 200 milligrams or less (in middle-aged adults). A level of just 240 would *double* that risk. So it is very important to be aware of your cholesterol level and to have it measured periodically. This is even more important if you have a family history of heart disease, or if you have one or more of the risk factors, such as high blood pressure or smoking.

These numbers are relative to age, by the way. A person in his eighties doesn't need to be as aggressive in lowering his cholesterol as a thirty-year-old, but both should try to get it down to normal levels.

Women should be aware that their cholesterol level may be 15 percent higher just before a menstrual period than during ovulation. Also, I recommend against getting a cholesterol check done in a shopping mall, where the methodology may be questionable.

The best ways to reduce cholesterol are to cut down on fatty and cholesterol-laden foods, to start exercising, and to stop smoking. Even vegetable oils, which contain no cholesterol, can raise the levels of LDL by causing the liver to manufacture more cholesterol to transport the excess fat. Also, limit your consumption of caffeine and alcohol, because they may raise your cholesterol level. A maximum of two cups of coffee and two alcoholic beverages a day is what you should strive for.

MY LOVED ONE HAS HEART DISEASE.
WHAT CAN I DO TO HELP?

Certainly you can encourage your loved one to exercise, eat sensibly, and learn to relax. I also feel it is important for family members to be prepared for any emergency. Have the phone number of the doctor, the hospital, and the ambulance right by the phone. You should be aware of the warning signs of heart attack. You should also learn how to do cardiopulmonary resuscitation (CPR). You can find instruction in this technique at the Red Cross or some Y's.

WHAT ARE THE SYMPTOMS
OF A HEART ATTACK?

The warning signals of a heart attack are usually a sense of severe pressure, generally in the center of the chest, which lasts for more than half an hour and frequently for several hours. The pressure may be experienced as a crushing pain or severe tightness. Sometimes pain may radiate to the arms, shoulders, or neck. The pain is usually accompanied by profound weakness, light-headedness, profuse sweating, and sometimes by nausea and difficulty in breathing.

These are the most common signs of heart attack. But there are other warnings as well. Here are some of the ways my patients have described the experience:

• "It was a burning sensation in my chest, like swallowing a spoonful of hot soup."
• "I felt nauseous and dizzy, and I was sweating profusely. I thought I had the flu."
• "It was a cramp in my back, and I felt real hot, like I was going to pass out."

SHOULD I TAKE EXTRA VITAMINS?

There is growing evidence that vitamin-rich diets can help prevent a variety of diseases, including heart disease. Recent studies have focused on the protective effects of the so-called antioxidant vitamins, which include vitamin C, vitamin E, and beta-carotene, which is related to vitamin A. Antioxidants protect us from free radicals, unstable atoms that can attack and destroy the chemical bonds in our bodies, leading to impaired immune function and degenerative changes, predisposing us to illness. Free radicals cannot be avoided. They are generated by sunshine, pollution, smoking, even exercise. But antioxidants bind with these free radicals, neutralizing them. It is believed, but not proved, that antioxidants somehow delay the oxidation of free radicals in the arterial wall, thus preventing or slowing the buildup of plaque.

Recent studies presented at the American Heart Association have shown that women who ate plenty of fruits and vegetables cut their risk of stroke by 54 percent, while men with similar diets were 30 percent less likely to die of heart disease. Other studies have found similar results. In the Harvard Nurses Study, those nurses who took supplements of vitamin E had less incidence of heart attack.

The antioxidant vitamins and some protective minerals, including zinc, chromium, and selenium, are widely available in food. Green, leafy vegetables and orange- and yellow-colored vegetables and fruits provide the most of these helpful substances. For extra protection, and with your doctor's advice, you might also want to take a multivitamin. Naturally, prevention of risk factors (low-fat diet, stopping smoking, and so on) is still the most important step you can take to protect your heart.

I'VE HEARD THAT FISH OIL IS
GOOD FOR YOUR HEART.

Fish oil contains polyunsaturated fatty acids known as omega-3 fatty acids. Experimental studies have demonstrated that people who consume these fats have fewer heart attacks. It is not known exactly how they work, but they seem to reduce the blood's tendency to clot.

Good sources of omega-3 fatty acids are salmon, trout, mackerel, sardines, herring, and bluefish. But be aware that some of these fish, such as bluefish, live in polluted coastal waters and should not be eaten too often. Bear in mind also that you will reverse the positive effects of the omega-3s if you fry the fish or serve it with a rich sauce. It is far better to broil or grill it.

Although supplements of omega-3 fatty acids are available in capsule form, they are high in calories and their long-term effects are unknown. I would recommend taking them only with the advice of a physician.

DOES OAT BRAN REALLY PROTECT
AGAINST HEART DISEASE?

We have known for a long time that oatmeal, as well as wheat bran, barley, beans, and peas, is a beneficial addition to the diet. All these food items, plus fruits and vegetables, contain fiber, which is important to the body in many ways: It helps keep the bowels functioning well, helps keep weight down, and can lower cholesterol. The best fibers for lowering cholesterol are those that are water soluble, such as oat bran.

I recommend adding as much fiber as possible to your diet, but be sure to read labels. One brand of oat bran muffins I saw in the supermarket contained twelve grams of fat!

CAN CLOT-DISSOLVING DRUGS
SAVE MY LIFE?

As we've already seen, most heart attacks are caused by a blood clot blocking a narrowed coronary artery. The damage to the heart results when its blood supply is cut off, so any way to restore the blood supply immediately should minimize or reduce the seriousness of the attack.

Modern medicine has come up with agents that can actually break up the blood clot that is causing the problem. They are called thrombolytic agents, and they include streptokinase, urokinase, and tissue plasminogen activator, or TPA. These chemicals, when administered intravenously or directly into the coronary artery, can reopen the artery.

Naturally, these drugs have the highest success rate when given within the first three hours after a heart attack begins, which is another reason it is vitally important to seek medical help if you have chest pains or other symptoms of heart attack.

Chapter Thirteen

LEARNING TO SMELL

THE FLOWERS

Mind your health; it's the most precious gift you have.
—Motto of Mind Your Health wellness and preventive health seminars

I have noticed that following a heart attack there is often a transformation. Some patients change their approach to life completely. They are usually calmer. They take more time with things. I believe that, having been so close to death, they have discovered what life is. They have learned to live in the moment.

But suppose you have not had that experience. I propose the following experiment: Close your eyes and pretend you are in the hospital with a heart attack. You are now confined to a bed, you are told everything you can and cannot do, you are even told when to go to the bathroom. You have to have intravenous drugs and oxygen; you have to stay in bed, immobilized.

A series of tests await you. Numerous blood samples will be taken.

Thoughts come into your mind, such as, Will I survive? Will I be able to see my children grow up? What if I can't go back to work? How long will I live? What will my friends say? What will happen to my family? You are told you have to take medication for the rest of your life, stop smoking, lose weight, follow a diet.

Why me? you wonder. I have so many things to do. So much is unfinished. These and similar thoughts cloud your mind. But then you reopen your eyes and realize that nothing has happened to you. You have the gift of health. You can do anything you want, go anywhere you like, and become anyone you really want to be. How marvelous! Everything is available to you.

Why wait until you have a heart attack to live this way? Why not live your life fully now? Health is a gift from God. It is a natural gift. Be aware of it and protect it. Enjoy and live life to the fullest *now*.

Why don't we all do this? I think it is at least partly because in our society pleasure is often regarded as a selfish pursuit. We feel that it is not as important as work. Yet the key element in health is not blood pressure, or cholesterol, or blood sugar. Instead, it is peace of mind and the ability to enjoy life. Indeed, this ability has been proved to prevent illness.

THE SECRETS OF TYPE B BEHAVIOR

Earlier in the book, I talked about Type A behavior, the hurry disease that is often coupled with anger and hostility. Far more healthy is Type B behavior, which can be learned. The hallmarks of this type of behavior include self-assurance, self-motivation, and the ability to relax in the face of pressures.

Just as the Type A person is aggressive and hostile, struggling to achieve more and more in less and less time, the Type B person is self-assured. She is self-motivated; an actor, not a reactor. This person's day is lived in an orderly fashion, and there is enough time for everything. Nothing is rushed or improvised; everything is planned.

The key characteristic of a Type A person is insecurity, because he measures the value of his personality according to the number of his achievements. So peace of mind is secondary to accomplishments. His achievements in turn depend on many factors outside his control. No wonder he becomes hostile and aggressive! He is constantly competing or challenging other people.

The Type B person doesn't need to compete or display her achievements. She finds self-confidence in self-approval, not by achieving goals. In essence she shifts her attention from the world around her to herself.

Just as Type A behavior has a number of harmful physiological effects, such as increased blood pressure and heart rate, Type B behavior can help to slow metabolism and is better for the health of all your body.

Type B behavior can be learned. Like any skill, it becomes better with practice. Gradually you can exchange outer-directed goals for inner ones. In this chapter are a number of suggestions for ways to learn to enjoy life. The ultimate goal is to create a sense of self-confidence and a serene mind. It may seem hopeless now, but all it really requires is self-knowledge and awareness.

I think of Corinne, a busy mother of three who had a heart attack when she was only thirty-one. Once she recovered, she found the strength to change her life. From working full-time she went to working part-time. From keeping her house always immaculately clean, she learned to let it get a little messy, to put up with a little dust. "You don't have to do everything," she told me when she was fully recovered. "You see, my mom stayed home with us kids, so I was trying to do what she did plus work at the same time, and now I've learned that you can't do it all. You can't be everything to everybody. If it doesn't get done, then it doesn't get done." Corinne had learned a valuable lesson that we could all take to heart: Accept yourself, imperfections and all.

Raising Your Consciousness

One day I was sitting with my mother near a beach. There was a construction site that prevented me from seeing the gulf area. I invited my mother to walk with me past the construction, and suddenly the whole beach was unimpeded before our eyes. The sky had a deep blue color, there were a few sailing boats skimming the water in the distance, and there was a point where the sea and the sky joined. It was a beautiful, inspiring view, but until I stood up and moved beyond the obstacle that was obscuring it, I was not aware of it.

So it can be with life. Things do not exist until we become aware of them. It is like the difference between living in an apartment on the ground floor and taking the elevator up to the top. Suddenly you discover new realities and horizons that were unknown to you. Think of the elevator as your consciousness. The higher our consciousness, the higher the point of view from which we look at ourselves and the world around us.

Einstein was once asked, What is the most important question that a man can ask himself? He replied, Is the world a friendly place? In other words, how do you look at the world? Do you see people as ready to help you, loving, kind, and accommodating? Or are they all enemies, out to take advantage of you?

This fundamental perception may be the key to achieving serenity. Serenity is not a gift that we receive from somebody. It is an inner experience. A state of mind like serenity doesn't come suddenly. It is a work that reveals itself when you clear your mind of negative thinking, hostility, hate, and unforgivingness.

Your mind is like a computer. It gives out what you put into it. So feed your mind with thoughts of peace, love, and serenity, and that will be your experience.

Give yourself time to relax. Give yourself the time to do the things you enjoy. The only important number in life is the number of days that we are allowed to remain on this planet. So live fully these days and remember that, if you want to live a beautiful life, you must first live beautiful days.

BEING HAPPY

Happiness is different for everyone. But I know a number of things that can keep you from being happy. For example, identifying yourself only with what you do. I have to admit that I suffer from this. I think of myself as a cardiologist, and I tie my self-worth to how good a cardiologist I am. But it doesn't work. It's too limiting. It makes me only Bruno the cardiologist, not Bruno the person.

This is something we all tend to do, and the result is that our moods depend entirely on how the day went at work. Good work = good day; bad work = bad day.

A physician I know always smiles. One day I asked him what was the source of his happiness, and he told me, "I am alive, no? That's all I need. Every day," he went on, "when I wake up and I'm alive, I'm happy. I'm grateful for every day that I live."

I believe that the *perception* of happiness is everything, and that the knowledge of this is especially important to cardiac patients. After all, they may find many reasons not to be happy: a heart problem, apprehension about the future, money worries. But these are all outer things. The inside, the real spiritual person, is not affected.

I think of Benny, who in addition to his heart problems has diabetes and must have dialysis three times a week. Despite all these disadvantages, he is the most optimistic person I have known. I once asked him what he thought about during dialysis, how he kept his good mood. Benny just looked at me and smiled. "I don't think about it, to tell you the truth," he said. "When I feel bad in the morning, then just as soon as I go on the machine

I feel good." He paused. "I know I will never get any better, so I just don't think about it."

I then asked him how a man with so many severe health problems could remain so optimistic. "I don't know how I would explain that," Benny said. "I realize I can't do what I would like to do. Of course my age is against me and the poor circulation; I can't walk too far, I get tired too fast. So I just take it from day to day and forget what happened in the past." He paused and gave me another sunny smile. "Maybe tomorrow will bring a better day to me," he said. "Who knows?"

Getting the Most out of the Present Moment

Somewhere I read that life is what goes on while we make other plans. In truth, so many of us are so busy looking at either the past or the future that we ignore the present moment. The secret of health and happiness lies instead in living in and enjoying the present to the fullest extent.

Living in the present is, in a way, an act of faith. It demonstrates faith in a friendly universe that surrounds us. It also implies faith in ourselves, our ability to do what is needed when it is needed. It implies love for ourselves, love enough to do the things that are best for us.

Now is the only moment there is. The past is gone, and the future is still to come. If you doubt me, observe children at play. They are the best teachers of living in the present. The idea of the past or the future doesn't exist in a child's mind. All he or she wants to do is enjoy the present to the fullest.

I'm reminded of another exceptional heart patient, Jack, who is sixty-eight. He developed heart disease when he was in his early fifties and lost his wife not long afterward. Yet he never complains about his bad luck or worries about the past or the future. "If I can live," he told me one day, "I want to live." Jack is active in his church and has many friends. When I asked him how he achieved such remarkable peace of mind, he shrugged. "I just take it as it comes," he told me. "I don't let things bother me. I think you should just get out and enjoy life, do things that you like to do."

Taking an Inventory of Life's Pleasures

I was lying under a tree enjoying the breeze and the shade during a hot summer day when it came to me that I always wanted to have a tree of my own and now I have one. This tree is beautiful and majestic. It is tall, slender, straight. I rest peacefully under it as if I were embraced by nature, relaxing in her arms and knowing that the tree is a shield for me, a safe place to be in. Lying down under that tree, I understood that in that place I had the opportunity to look inside and sense the beauty of the moment. I was happy then. This was one of my life pleasures. Just being myself and realizing that I had all I needed to be happy.

I began then to think of all the other pleasures in my life, all the simple and not so simple things that let me be myself and express my own happiness. I had never before thought to take an inventory of life's pleasures, but I now see the value of doing just that. Most of us, including me, are concerned most of the time about how to avoid pain rather than how to gain pleasure. When we are children, our parents and other authority figures are always warning us that life is not simple. They tell us to be careful, to avoid this and that.

But as we become more aware of what our satisfactions are, it will be easier to acknowledge and enjoy them. There are many diversions that make me happy. Sports, for instance. Have you ever had the fun of windsurfing? All you need is a board and a sail. You stand up on the board and let the wind carry you. It is beautiful to feel the wind on your body, the water under your feet. You feel light, agile, and in touch with nature. When the wind isn't strong, you can enjoy the surroundings, the people, the blue sky, and savor this moment of letting go.

I have many other pleasures. One of my life's greatest pleasures is self-expression, which I fulfill by writing in my journal. Becoming aware of God within me and finding inner peace are to me very gratifying. My family is a great source of joy to me. I draw pleasure from talking to my wife and listening to her poetry. I draw pleasure from listening to and advising my children, Veronica and Maximillian. It is fulfilling for me to read, especially on the themes of spirituality and self-empowerment. I also love public speaking because to me, to touch people's hearts and help them change their lives for the better is one of the greatest joys.

Many of my exceptional heart patients have learned to be aware of and value the pleasures in their lives. One who comes to mind is Nick, who had a heart attack in his early sixties. Nick owns an upholstery shop and had always been very active, despite severe arthritis. After the heart attack he was forced to curtail his activities, especially sports. But he wasn't fazed. He simply switched to other pleasures. "I've always been someone who appreciates a challenge," Nick told me. "And I'm not going to give up. I find a lot of enjoyment out of little things in life. Why worry about the fact that I can't play basketball or I can't be active in that regard? I enjoy certain TV programs. I enjoy reading. I enjoy just visiting with friends. I enjoy all those little things that I can do, just sitting out front on a beautiful sunny day or watching the leaves turn. What [the heart attack] has done for me is make me appreciate the small things in life. You don't need a lot of outside stimulation to make you happy."

What about you? Where do you find your greatest joys?

Take a moment now to jot down the things that give you pleasure. They might be as simple and common as smelling a rose or as complicated as building a ship in a bottle. Try to list them all. Later on when additional things occur to you, add them to the list. Then take time each day to fulfill at least some of the desires on the list.

Adding to Your Pleasures

You probably already know many of the activities that give you pleasure. But maybe you have been a workaholic. Maybe you never did take time out to smell the roses, time for yourself and your own happiness. I'm going to give you some suggestions for pleasures that many of my exceptional heart patients have enjoyed and that you can make your own.

JOURNALING. Keeping a daily journal not only is enriching but also can help you in your spiritual journey. You don't have to write a lot, but it's a good idea to spend at least five minutes, to write a little every day. As for what to write about, that's up to you. Write what you're feeling, what you did today, what your hopes and fears are for the future. Write about what you would like to be doing. Write about someone you love or someone from your past that you miss.

Being honest with yourself in a journal is an excellent way to diffuse feelings and to discover the assumptions underneath them. It will help you get to know yourself better.

GARDENING. Gardening can be ideal for cardiac patients because it totally absorbs your attention. This focusing can allow you to forget your problems. Also, gardening is usually done outdoors, where you can breathe fresh air. It can put you in touch with nature and remind you of the commonality of all living things, bringing you closer to God. Seeing a flower in its perfection is a way of acknowledging the infinite intelligence that surrounds us.

My own experience with gardening is limited, but I always remember one incident in particular. When a friend of mine learned that my sister had died in Italy, he brought me a small plant and said, "Why don't you plant this in your garden? Then every day as you water it and it grows, the plant will remind you of your sister."

I did as he advised and still have that plant, now a beautiful flowering bush. It does remind me of my sister. Metaphorically, I believe that plants are like ideas. If we have an idea and keep focusing on it—feeding that idea daily with our enthusiasm, hopes, dreams, and will to grow—it will grow.

CULTIVATING HOUSEPLANTS. If for whatever reason you can't garden outdoors, do the next best thing and grow plants indoors. Not only do indoor plants look attractive but they are natural antipollutants that help to clear the air of smoke and other toxins. In addition, several houseplants in a room can help reduce the noise level. Houseplants also make people feel calmer and more optimistic. One study has shown that hospital patients whose rooms faced a garden recovered more quickly and better than those whose rooms faced a wall.

KEEPING PETS. The physical and emotional benefits of keeping pets are well known. Just interacting with a pet can result in lowered blood pressure and heart rate, and general decrease of stress. Pets are nonjudgmental and give us their unconditional love. By sharing our feelings with them, we make pets our intimate friends, bonding with them strongly.

A study on heart attack victims at the University of Pennsylvania, reported in *Pet Love* by Betty White, demonstrated that owning a pet made a significant difference in survival. Apparently dealing with animals refocuses our attention from our own worries, reducing stress and anxiety. In addition, the need to exercise pets gives us an opportunity to remain active.

I've always been close to pets. When I was a child, I had a dog who was my companion, confidant, and playmate. These days we own a cockatoo that was given to my daughter. I find this bird exceptionally intelligent. As soon as I open the door, the bird starts singing, and then, if the door to his cage is open, he flies and lights on my shoulder, continuously chirping, showing me his great joy in being with me. Sometimes I think how beautiful life would be if we all had on our shoulder someone or something that was chirping and creating good humor.

It is true that pets can sometimes be demanding, but I firmly feel that the love we give to them is abundantly returned. We are never too old to own a pet. Elderly people in particular seem to benefit. If they become sick, having a pet to care about seems to speed their recovery. Also, because so many of the elderly live alone, owning a pet is a good way for them to alleviate their loneliness, as well as to increase their sense of security.

ENJOYING HEAT AND RELAXATION. Hot water has a beneficial effect on the mind and body. It reduces tension and relaxes muscles. It is especially good for heart patients because it dilates blood vessels and increases circulation. I am speaking here of moderately hot water, of course, not extremely hot, which can cause the heart to beat faster and work harder. If you have access to a hot tub or spa, or even a hot bath, soak in it to unwind at the end of the day. For safety's sake, limit your bathing to no more than fifteen or twenty minutes.

Saunas too can be very relaxing, as can steam baths. The steam bath, in fact, was used by Hippocrates, the father of medicine, in his cures. Whereas the sauna provides a high-temperature, low-humidity environment, the steam bath provides high moisture as well as heat, which can be beneficial to the skin.

There are, of course, many, many other things that can bring pleasure: playing chess, holding a baby, collecting stamps or coins—choose whatever you like. Don't put it off because you are too busy or don't want to "waste" time on frivolous activities. Nothing is frivolous if it contributes to your happiness and well-being.

HAVING A SENSE OF HUMOR. Answering machine: "You have reached the office of Dr. Spritz. If you have chest pain, press 1. If you have shortness of breath, press 2. If you feel awful, press 3. And if you are using a rotary dial phone, hang up. You can't afford Dr. Spritz." This joke just goes to illustrate that we can't take ourselves too seriously all the time. And this is especially so when we are sick. As Norman Cousins demonstrated in *Anatomy of an Illness*, laughter can literally save your life.

Yet too many of us, I think, avoid humor and laughter. We think it is silly or frivolous. We definitely avoid it on the job. I notice this a lot among physicians. I seldom see them laughing. Most of the time, in fact, physicians are affected by chronic seriousness. Patients, too, aren't supposed to laugh, because if you laugh it means you are well. If you are well, you don't belong in a physician's office. This is a paradox that keeps both participants in the patient-physician relationship from relaxing. A little laughter would be so helpful to both.

It's not always easy to be lighthearted and laugh, but if you can see the humor in everything, you will be able to recover more quickly. I will never forget John, a retired professor who needed bypass surgery. The surgeon told me that everyone in the operating room burst into laughter when John was wheeled in. There, taped to his chest, was a carefully drawn diagram of the heart and circulatory system with his affected artery outlined in red!

HEARTSKILL 8: FEELING-LIFE INVENTORY

The following inventory is designed to help you become acquainted with your feeling patterns, so that you can learn what affects you positively and what affects you negatively. Your answers should give you a rough idea of what you really *feel* you need to be comfortable and happy. It will also show where you do and don't *feel* you are getting those needs met at the present time, and, in some cases, how you are acting on the feeling patterns you operate with now.

1. What is your first feeling as you realize you are awake in the morning? What is your second feeling?

2. Outside of hygiene, what are the first five steps in your morning routine? Why do you include them and place them in that order?

3. If you could drop five "required" activities from your life, what would they be and why would you drop them?

4. What "treats" do you have tucked away for special or emergency occasions? What about these treats makes them work for you?

5. Who do you live, work, or associate with who gets under your skin? What comes up inside you when you think about dropping that person from your life?

6. Look over a list of your family members, friends, business associates, and acquaintances. Who are you jealous of? What is the jealousy about?

7. You have a magic wand and right now can change anything you want to about your body, living situation, work and leisure time. What would you change and why?

8. Who would you rather die than confront? Why? About what?

9. How would you describe your best friend?

10. You have died. How do you feel about what your obituary says about you?

Evaluating Your Feeling-Life Inventory

Many people honestly don't know their requirements for happiness. I believe that this is partly because thinking of one's own happiness is somehow considered selfish, and also because many of us simply settle for what is rather than strive to achieve what might be. In any case, the answers to your feeling-life inventory can help you become acquainted—perhaps for the first time— with the things and attitudes that make you most comfortable and happy, as well as with those things that detract from your happiness.

Your answer to Question 1 reveals your overall outlook on your life at present. Ideally, you should experience positive feelings first thing in the morning. If this is not true—if, for example, you think, "Oh, no, another day at the job"—this is a sign that your job is not providing you with the support you need. Likewise, if you wake up feeling tired, or with a cigarette cough, this is a message from your body that the things you are doing are not promoting health and happiness for you.

Question 2 relates most strongly to your health habits: Of the five items you listed, how many are supporting your good health and well-being? Examples of such activities include exercise, stretching, meditation, eating breakfast. If, on the other hand, your early morning activities are negative, such as lighting a cigarette or drinking coffee to "clear the cobwebs," you should try to change some of these habits to more positive ones.

Questions 3 and 4 refer to activities that may be contributing to any emotions or bad feelings you experience. While some unpleasant activities—such as a job you dislike—cannot be dropped from your life without considerable thought and planning, others, such as chairing a tiresome co-op board meeting, can be eliminated with less difficulty than you might expect. Carefully look over your list of unwanted activities and try to eliminate—or minimize—as many of them as you can.

Likewise, review your list of special treats and stop using them only for "emergency" purposes; try instead to incorporate at least one of them in your life every day or so. If you can't think of five treats now, make it a point to discover some.

Questions 5 and 6 relate to the people in your life who may cause unhappy feelings from time to time. If someone inevitably causes you anxiety, it might be a good idea to drop that person from your life if doing so is possible. If it's not (if, for example, that person is your boss), try to find out why that person makes you feel bad. Does he or she remind you of a bossy parent? Of the parts of yourself that you dislike? Sometimes understanding the reasons for unpleasant interactions can help to resolve them. Jealousy, on the other hand, is often a key to your own unmet inner needs. Examine any jealous feelings you have and try to determine why you have them. Do you envy another's health, for example, or large circle of friends? If so, it is time to work on improving your own health or expanding your own social circle.

Question 7, the magic wand question, can be a kind of magic wand itself if you take action on the answer you gave: Begin now to change the things that you are unhappy with—or at least begin to work toward changing them. Remember that although you can seldom change outward circumstances, you can *always* change your feelings about them.

Not everyone will have an answer to Question 8, though all of us have acquaintances and family members who we feel uncomfortable confronting. If you actually cannot confront someone, I suggest sitting in a quiet spot and imagining the confrontation, in as much detail as you can manage. Very often this simple exercise will put a conflict to rest.

Question 9, about your best friend, is a strong indication of the personality traits that make you most happy. Even if your friend upsets you from time to time, it is his or her positive traits that drew you together. Try to cultivate these traits in yourself.

As with Question 7, Question 10 can be acted on immediately. If you're not sure what changes you would like to make, try writing your ideal obituary, and begin taking steps now to make it come true.

Chapter Fourteen

CREATING YOUR FUTURE

———————

*We have something within us that is
greater than we are.*
—Carleton Whitehead

The heart is seen in different ways by different people. We physicians look at it as a pump that keeps human beings alive, delivering oxygen and nutrients to vital organs and throughout the body. For us, then, the heart is the center station from which all circulation originates and is maintained, but it is still a muscle—or, as a transplant surgeon I know once said, "a stupid muscle."

How can he say that? I wondered at the time. Because for me the heart is so much more. Traditionally, the heart has been thought to be the site of the soul. It is also the center of love, as well as of negative feelings such as hate, hostility, revenge, and denial.

I believe that the heart has a memory and an infinite intelligence within it, and I can't think of any organ that is closer to the mind than the heart. As physicians, we received training geared to believing only in what we can cut and see, in the materialistic view of the world. Yet the work of the heart is in part still beyond our understanding.

I prefer to think of the heart as the center of love, and I can imagine the emptiness of a heart which is devoid of this fundamental principle that keeps us united to one another with an infinite power.

Is your heart empty or is it full? If it is full, what does it contain? No one can judge you. No one can see within you. It can certainly be helpful to examine the fullness of your heart and consciously ascertain that it is what you want to express in your life. Ideally, the content of the heart is love, peace, joy, happiness, and creativity. It is also the spiritual sparkle that breathes into every cell of the body.

What if your heart has been wounded by heart disease or a heart attack? It is still the same. I look at the heart as a spiritual organ, so even the physically wounded heart is spiritually perfect. Looking at it this way, a positive result of heart disease is the certain knowledge that you are not immortal, and that you have the opportunity to plan for a more worthwhile, fulfilling life.

CHOOSING YOUR OWN PATH
TO CONTENTMENT

Many believe that the purpose of life is to find out why we are on this planet. This is another way of saying that one of life's drives is toward goals. Having a goal means having a destination. Having a destination means making plans and then taking action to reach that destination.

We all need goals. Without goals there is no life. Goals help us to channel our energy, mobilize our creativity, and focus it into something meaningful. When I speak of goals I mean all sorts: personal goals, family goals, social goals. As we create our goals, we also create a hierarchy of values, because goals, in my opinion, are based upon values. So another way of examining one's goals is to ask, What do I value the most?

Some people codify their goals by writing them down and then reviewing them from time to time. It is important to be clear what values, what goals you hold. Whether or not you actually achieve the goal, what is important is what you become in order to achieve it. Becoming is more important than having. Goals give you a sense of purpose, meaning, and direction. A life without goals is a life not fully lived.

Exceptional Heart Patients

On a recent trip I had the privilege of meeting with Dr. Dean Ornish. He has dedicated his life to a dream, proving that heart disease can improve and even be reversed with diet, exercise, and behavioral changes. When we open our hearts to spirituality, miracles take place, and Dean has been able to demonstrate scientifically the validity of this truth. I spent one afternoon with Dean's patients and discovered how exceptional they are. They are people who had the courage to say no to a verdict of invalidism or inevitably deteriorating coronary disease. These people had the courage to embrace Dean Ornish's philosophy of life and put it into action. And each of them saw his or her symptoms subside daily.

I especially remember Francis, who had refused immediate surgery. "I am competent," he told me. "I prefer to be responsible for my own health. I can take care of my body." Now, four years later, he was symptom-free and enjoying the fruits of Dr. Ornish's program of daily exercise, sensible diet, and meditation.

I was so happy during the time I spent with these patients. Each of them had a special enthusiasm, a joy for life, that was contagious. They had taken charge of their own lives and changed them. I was also captivated by Dean's own spirituality and gentleness. Here was a man who had a goal that he had turned into a miracle.

I want to emphasize here that while Dr. Ornish created his program, it is his patients who are daily living the goals. The choice is always with you, to make health your own goal. I used to be upset when a patient would not follow my orders. But I gradually grew into the idea that each patient has a mind of his own, a will of her own, and it is my job not to obstruct that will but rather to understand and support it. This is even more true if the situation is serious. Let's say I believe cardiac catheterization is needed and the patient refuses. I say, "Look, I told you that your condition needs to be investigated. The pains you are having are the heart's way of talking to you. Please, listen to that signal. Don't ignore it." But if the patient chooses not to listen to me, I respect that decision. I have done my job, and I am at peace. No matter what the patient does, I will not deprive her or him of my love.

Of course, like all doctors, I want to see concrete, physical results of healing. But to tell you the truth, *when* the patient is healed is sometimes debatable. Healing can take place in mysterious ways. Healing of the heart and soul is more meaningful than the outward evidence of health. Who can tell us that physical healing is more important than spiritual?

It comes back to goals. What is the most important value to each patient? I think over and over of my exceptional heart patients, and how each of them set different goals. The most important goal was surviving or continuing to love life.

When most of these patients were in the coronary care unit recovering from their heart attacks or other heart problems, they got in touch with the deepest part of themselves. From that inner self they drew the courage and strength to decide to continue to live, even to fight for their lives. They decided to overcome disease and walk again in the pathway of health. That required considerable effort in many cases, but these spiritual giants were able to do it successfully.

I have long been inspired by these patients and have spoken to many of them about their further goals after survival. Not surprisingly, for most of them, the second goal was to live for love of the family. Then, having left the hospital, their third major step toward recovery was to resume work. I think work is often overlooked as a component of recovery, but the truth is that our work gives us dignity as human beings. It is proof that we are contributing to life, making the world a better place in which to live.

Finally, for nearly all patients, there was a goal of a closer union with God, however God was defined. Whether this meant developing a higher level of spirituality or getting in touch with the divinity within, this spiritual element was a vital part in the recovery of most of these patients.

Sylvia is a shining example of someone who used her goals to pull her through a most difficult time. Sick with cardiomyopathy, Sylvia had a heart transplant in her mid-thirties. The difficult operation and periods of rejection of the new heart might have stopped a lesser person. But Sylvia clung to her goals. "Even when I was the sickest," she told me, "I realized that it was important to never give up my dream and to have hope. I tried always to have a goal for the day, even if it was as simple as just eating all my meals. So I would wake up every morning knowing what I wanted to get done. I think it is very important to set a goal for yourself. Long-range goals are also important to keep you going. Like for me, my daughter's graduation, but it could be anything you've planned and hoped for."

Daniel, a lifelong athlete, had been experiencing increasing shortness of breath and had lost the sight in his right eye. I encouraged him to resume exercise and start meditation, keeping in mind his goals for a more healthy life. He took my advice, and his life changed! Not only has he been able to resume his favorite sport of archery but he is now an instructor for the Junior Olympic Archery Team.

MY GOALS FOR A MORE HUMAN MEDICINE

I have stated before that I believe modern medicine is in the midst of an amazing transformation, and one of my personal goals is to take part in that transformation. I want to help facilitate the conversion of our system to a more human, spiritual, and love-based medicine.

I try to live my goals each day by teaching my patients how to be healthy and by loving them unconditionally. I see myself not as dealing with disease, as I and all doctors were taught, but rather as dealing with people who *have* disease. I envision a day when physicians see their primary role as educators: teaching people how to be well. After all, we become doctors primarily to help people. The patient seeks the feeling of love in the physician's eyes. The patient needs to sense that he or she is loved and cared for. One of the most gratifying and rewarding experiences I recall is when a patient told me, "You are not just a doctor, you are my friend."

I also envision a day when the patient is a full partner in health care. When patients understand the intimate connection between body and mind, and strive actively for health of both body and soul. I foresee the day when all physicians extend our collaboration with patients to the point where we understand their consciousness and inner worlds and don't limit ourselves to the superficial aspects of disease.

I am beginning to share my ideas on other changes, including a transformation of our nation's hospitals. The way things are today, I don't think that many hospitals are the ideal place to recover, at least for those categories of disease, such as heart disease, where both mind and body are involved. In some hospitals, for example, there is no way to see the sun, no flowers, no children laughing. There is essentially no life. I'm sure you've been in some of these hospitals, big concrete blocks with narrow corridors, the loudspeaker always squawking, and patients languishing in tiny, dark rooms with windows that look out on an airshaft or a parking lot.

The truth is that the patient is the main source of livelihood for the hospital, and the patient's joy and pleasant stay should be of supreme importance to the hospital staff. In the hospital of the future, the personnel should visit with the patient more attentively and with utmost care. They should ask if she needs an extra blanket at night, ask him, in essence, what can be done to please him. There should be people available who speak several languages, and all should be trained in humane, human contact.

Rather than the sterile, boxy buildings of today, I dream of hospitals that have glass ceilings, where you can see the sky, hear the rain, smell the flowers. Where you can walk outdoors, under the trees. I dream of hospitals with soundproof rooms to scream or weep in. Where hugging therapeutics are mandatory three or four times daily, and where lessons in loving oneself and others are given. If I as a doctor am skilled enough to heal your disease, after all, why don't I go even further and help you to improve your overall health, not just of body but of soul?

FINDING YOUR OWN MEANING IN LIFE AND DEATH

I've been reading some books on death and dying, and as I read I find I have to ask myself certain questions. Even though I feel in perfectly good health, how would I react to being told that I had six months to live? The first thing that comes to mind is how many things I have left undone. I want to see my grandchildren grown up. I want to enjoy life more. All these years I've been focusing on work, work, work, and trying to gain financial security. I'd love to enjoy the company of my wife and children, friends, see the world and really enjoy success.

On the other hand, like all of us, I sometimes have down

periods when I don't love myself enough or accept my limitations. Often I let my life be driven by others. I don't always have the courage to declare that I, too, am in need of love, that there are parts of my personality I don't accept. As physicians, we can too often forget that our patients have the same ambivalence about life and death.

I dislike having to give bad news to patients. I try to do the best I can in my daily practice, so that the patients leaving the office somehow feel better than when they first came. But sometimes it is difficult not to discourage them. I have to make a conscious effort to tell the real truth without adding a sugar coating. On the other hand, I don't want to give a death sentence or statistics that are discouraging and disempowering.

Despite my belief that there is a part of us that lives beyond the body, there is no harder task for a physician than to realize a patient will soon die. It is in part because of our training: patient's death = doctor's failure. Also, it forces *us* to confront the reality of death. That is never more apparent than when we talk to the family, seeing the pearls of tears in their eyes. Yet at some point death is not in the hands of the doctor at all but of the patient.

Earlier in the book I spoke about how some patients seem to want to die. It is my experience that patients, when faced with the inevitable, are able to choose the moment and manner of their death. This may sound fantastic, but I have seen it happen over and over. Sometimes patients wait for the doctor, if there was an agreement to wait. I remember Annette, a cardiac patient with advanced heart failure. She was very close to the end of her life when I went out of town, but she waited for me to come back three days later. When I saw her, she was comatose. I kissed her, and about ten minutes later her heart slowed down and then stopped as she died peacefully. I believe that she waited for me.

Another patient, Virginia, a German lady of eighty-four with blue eyes, pale skin, and a very strong personality, survived a severe heart attack. True to her personality, she declined any special tests or studies. She came for a cardiac checkup three or four times a year, and actually did very well.

Then she became ill with intestinal cancer. Because of her previous heart attack and age, surgery was considered especially risky, and she refused it. She was put on tube feeding and transferred to the extended care unit in our hospital. In consultation between her and her children, we agreed to put "Do Not Resuscitate" on her chart.

Despite her extreme illness and progressive weakness, Virginia had the same request for me every day when I came to see her. "Doctor," she said, looking straight into my eyes, "I want to go home." Every day she would insist. "Can I go home today or tomorrow?" She was ready at any time.

Finally her family consented to take her back home. The day she left, I gave her a kiss. She was as thin as a concentration camp victim. I held her daughter and wished the best for her mother. Three days later the nurse called to tell me that Virginia had died peacefully at home, where she wanted to die.

HEARTSKILL 9:
SELF-ACCEPTANCE EXERCISE

The title of this Heartskill exemplifies my purpose in writing this book: to help others to heal their hearts by accepting themselves. In a sense we are all heart patients, if you define the heart as the center of soul, because anything that happens in our bodies or in our minds ultimately affects the heart. Further, since all of us need to heal some aspects of our personalities or behavior, this healing is lifelong.

I read somewhere that you only possess a thing if you can share it; if you can't share it then you don't own it.

Self-acceptance means literally that we accept ourselves just as we are. It means that we recognize ourself *independently* from our performance. To the degree that we do not accept ourselves, we reject ourselves.

The foundation of self-acceptance lies in the recognition that we are spiritual beings; this recognition eliminates the need to seek the approval and acceptance of others. To practice the heartskill of self-acceptance, take every opportunity to repeat to yourself:

> I accept myself.
> I appreciate myself.
> I respect myself.

This exercise is especially helpful if you say the words while looking at yourself in a mirror, even hugging yourself.

Afterword

THE HEART

OF A CARDIOLOGIST

Where do I come from? Why am I here? The answers to these existential questions are simple in my case. I am here because I choose to be here. My family comes from the small southern Italian town of Oristano. I was the fourth child of five, and besides the members of my immediate family I had many other loving relatives. I especially remember Aunt Amelia, who showed me how to love people and taught me to give to others. I was raised in Sardinia until I graduated from the University of Cagliari.

I had always been interested in medicine, so I became a physician, and during my studies I was attracted by the magic of the heart. I spent several years in Turin studying cardiology. I became a specialist and a professor, which had been one of my lifelong dreams, but for various reasons the teaching did not work out as I had hoped. I discovered that my values were not the same as the values of those I was working with, and that I did not have the political "push" it seemed to take to get ahead. I decided it was time for a complete change and moved to the United States, where I hoped my values would be respected.

I had earlier married an adorable medical student named Pia; soon Veronica and Maximillian came to keep us company, so now we had a family of four. We settled in Chicago, and Pia told me to open my own office. "See people," she said. "You are good with people." So I did, and my practice became a success with patients. But then I found myself missing the university experience, the give-and-take of meetings and seminars. I was doing research on laser surgery and traveled all over the world to present my studies, but though I enjoyed those moments, they were not really what I was looking for.

I enjoyed being a cardiologist, I liked to be able to extend someone's life by, say, performing a successful angioplasty. But there was a dark, less fulfilling side to my practice. For one thing, the large number of chronically ill patients, the repeaters, and other visible signs of traditional medicine's failure to address disease and suffering began to bother me. The ocean of paperwork, the intricate structure of medical and hospital politics forced me to see how medicine cripples itself. I became anxious and frustrated with the thought that my life seemed to be dedicated to waiting at the hospital for the next cardiac victim. What people really needed, I increasingly felt, was not to be sick in the first place.

Around this time I wrote in my journal: "I'm tired. Tired of seeing young people die of heart attacks. Tired of seeing the eyes of wives and children whose husbands and fathers never came home from the emergency room. Tired of seeing chests split open for surgery, or learning that someone else was brought in dead on arrival."

I was frustrated too by the lack of spirituality in modern medicine. It was as if the human body were just a collection of parts, rather than an organic, whole unified by an animating spirit.

Gradually I realized that I could invest all I had learned in some thirty years of practice toward health rather than disease.

At the same time my own interest shifted from the traditional physician's orientation to disease toward one of health. I then began to encourage my patients to share their feelings with me, and I began to share mine with them. I found that by dropping my professional mask, I had given myself an opportunity to discover my patients as people, and, in a way, my patients became my support group.

The more I experienced myself as a human being, the more I began to see my patients as such also. I learned to meet their eyes, to be warmer, more present, thoughtful, caring, and attentive to them. For example, one day I realized what a distance my office desk put between me and my patients during consultations. I decided to draw up a chair next to the patients instead and to record our interviews because their stories so moved me.

When I sensed that a patient was comfortable with a touch or could be helped by it, I began to give a pat on the arm, a squeeze around the shoulders, or even a big hug. Reaching out changed my world. I started to laugh with my patients, to cry with them, to spend time with them by choice—and to feel urgent about what more I could do to help them get well, stay well, live long lives.

So I was happy with my family, my research, my practice, but something was still missing. One day I found out what it was: I opened a new office, where I created a conference room for my patients. I felt a need to be closer, literally in touch with them. I realized that this was my opportunity to teach them what I have learned *before* they have to pay such a high price with their health; that their own minds can free them; that they have the power to heal themselves if they will assume personal responsibility for their health.

I realized that I could invest all I have learned in thirty years of practice toward health; that my life could still be dedicated to people but now in the realm of health. As I began to see this, the magic flame within me leapt with an excitement and hope that I had not experienced for a long time. Now my mission was becoming clear. My interest had shifted from the physician's orientation, disease, to health, and from patients to people. In that conference room I discovered the secret: *Our hearts are the same*.

THE MEDICINE OF LOVE

When I sat down with my patients and opened my heart to them, and they opened their hearts to me, we discovered the beauty of this relationship. To me, meeting with my patients in this setting was the greatest joy, the most fulfilling role I had played. I learned about them as humans, and they learned the same about me. I especially remember the night that my mask as a physician fell aside. I was still trying to grasp the things I had learned about myself and my profession in the course of my spiritual search. I had tears in my eyes as I told the men and women in that room about my realizations, how I had been hurting myself and others by hiding my true self. I told them how, by ruthlessly pursuing grown-up goals, I had made the child part of myself suffer unbearably. As I spoke, my patients leaned forward. I could see from their eyes that they were with me—not as a doctor but simply as a human being in terrible pain, trying to get his soul back.

That's when it happened—when I realized that, by sharing myself in my humanity, I was opening the way for my patients to do the same. This event tore down the artificial barrier between us. I understood then that I didn't have to do anything more than be myself, be their partner in healing. And I found that by sharing with them I also was healed.

From then on, in that conference room, my patients and I shared secrets, cried together, hugged each other. At last I was becoming aware of what I really wanted to do. My mission was to bring the principles of good health to others, to empower them in overcoming disease. Finally, I could talk about health and not disease.

I was choosing the freedom to be what I always wanted to be, a teacher. I began to work on creating a seminar to take my message to even more people, to touch even more hearts. In sharing the message, you see, I am not only a cardiologist but a man with a heart. My happiness has become the discovery of a purpose in life, finding out what, deep inside, I really wanted.

It may seem presumptuous, but I mean to do whatever I can in my practice to accomplish this goal. I don't know how much I am going to accomplish; all I know is that I feel good doing it. It is in harmony with myself and the world around me.

This is the reason for this book.

My roles as a teacher and writer are still in their infancy. They are a beginning for me on this new path. Taking up this direction is a spiritual action for me, and its benefits cannot help but show up in my health, exactly as the same action must for anyone.

Spirituality has changed my life. The discovery that I can have the consciousness of God, see God in everyone I meet, and desire to touch people's hearts brings me to the conclusion that there is a priest in every physician—not just a remnant of the witch doctor or shaman but a priest in the sense of a person who can build a bridge to God for another. I believe that God is within each of us. This knowledge of the divinity within is a pathway to health through personal development. I know now that health depends on self-discovery and spiritual attunement, and is realized through loving others and sharing yourself with them.

I hope that my words have touched your heart, and that you will begin to move to heal your own heart and soul. I'd like to leave you with the words of a prayer/poem that came to me while I was meditating one day.

The Eyes of God

When you see through the eyes of God, you see only beauty and perfection around you.

When you see through the eyes of God, other people become you.

When you see through the eyes of God, you accept yourself, all of yourself,

And discover the purpose of life: to become all that you are.

Then, only then, you are free, you are pure love

Seeing through the eyes of God.

Appendix

HOPE AND THE CARDIAC
PATIENT:
A NOTE FOR HEALTH
PROFESSIONALS

---

would not have written this book if I did not love my work as a cardiologist. After all, angioplasty and other procedures allow me to change the course of people's lives. To be able to be of service in such a way is more satisfying than I know how to say. My desires to prevent death before its natural time, to share my love for humanity in ways that really make a difference, are as great today as they were when I entered medical school.

But what I have learned through my years of practice is that the physician's job goes far beyond the technical aspects of diagnosis and treatment. I believe that in some ways our most important challenge is to encourage elements of hope in the patient's mind. The truth is that for cardiac patients, or for any other patients, hope is an essential ingredient in recovery, and the physician has great power to enhance hope. The enhancement of hope has to be honest, however—it is wrong to raise false hope. The physician's real job, then, is to help the patient live realistically with his or her own illness.

This is not as easy as it may sound, because unfortunately we physicians have been trained to deal only with the disease—in a word, the facts. Anything beyond the material world, outside the confines of what can be measured, we have been trained to stay out of because these things are what we call soft data.

Yet I am convinced that such intangible elements are just as real as hard data such as blood pressure numbers. More important, they are just as essential—even more so—to our patients' recovery. Why is it that some people die prematurely while others live long beyond their expected time of survival? I believe hope is an element in these circumstances. I have personally seen that hope and faith play a major role in patient recovery and well-being.

Hope is a shield against fear. It's an interaction between the patient and the physician, rather than something material that can be given. When the patient looks into the physician's eyes, he or she is seeking that element of hope. Hope and love are first cousins.

We physicians are in a special position to help patients by increasing their hope. On the other hand, sometimes we can kill hope and thus hasten the end of lives. More than once I have become so absorbed by the medical data that I have been ready to leave a patient's room without any human interaction until I've been stopped by the patient's appeal, "So, Doc, how am I doing?" Only then have I realized that my thoughts at that moment were channeled toward classic medicine and not toward the patient. I was more concerned about the appropriateness of the diagnostic test or the ramifications of the diagnosis than about the patient's desperate need to know what was going on.

Simple communication of reassurance can build hope in patients. When hope is thus enhanced, patients become more self-confident. They trust their hearts more; they are able to face confidently the difficulties and opportunities that lie ahead. The element of hope can channel the strength and determination to continue cardiac rehabilitation, to keep on losing weight, to stop smoking, to follow a new diet, ultimately to take care of one's own heart.

How do we convey this hope?

I think of one patient who is seventy-five years old, in really incredible physical shape. Even after open-heart surgery he still jogs and plays tennis. One day after an examination he looked me in the eye and said, "Doc, whenever I come here and I hear your words, they really push me up and give me greater courage. I feel fantastic leaving this office." I tried to think what I had done and then realized how I encourage him: "Don't pay any attention to what people say about your age," I tell him. "You look fantastic to me, and I have many eighteen-year-olds who would not be able to keep up with you." Every word I say is true—and how easy it is to say them. But how easy it would be not to say anything, to keep our interaction on a purely businesslike basis.

Another part of building hope is letting patients know what is possible. I remember Gerald, who suffered from congestive heart failure. He came to me saying, "I was stressed by my cardiologist. She didn't understand me. My heart was oversized and pumping inefficiently." I encouraged him to start an exercise program. "I decided," he told me, "to take charge of my life; I studied nutrition and did my own searching. I feel I am regenerating my body exercising every day and meditating. I use this affirmation, 'My heart is beating in perfect coordination with the healing rhythm of the universe.' "

With Gerald I didn't add any new technical treatments, all I did was introduce the element of hope and let him know that it was possible for him to do something for his own heart, to help heal it and keep it in good shape. He might have already known this on an intellectual level from his reading, but I believe that hearing it from his physician made the difference. The truth is that even the best-informed patient often looks for advice from the physician in order to gain a sense of security.

A further element of hope, for me, is to mention to patients who are receptive that their essence is not just body but also spirit, and that the healing of the physical heart depends on the healing of the spiritual heart. I think that giving patients this perspective can raise their consciousness beyond the purely materialistic view that life is linked to the physical condition of the heart and that an unhealthy heart is automatically a death sentence.

Hope is conveyed not just in words but also in attitude, in communicating that you care. According to Dr. Ronna Jevne, author of *No Time for Nonsense*, hope is manifested in the way you look at the patient, in your smile, in the tone of your voice, in your body language, in sitting and holding the patient's hands, in hugging the patient when she is low in spirit, and in letting the patient know that you have been there, that you have faced difficult times too.

Another way I try to give hope is to encourage patients with stories of other patients who have overcome adversity. I tell them about my exceptional heart patients, such as the eighty-one-year-old man who, after two angioplasties, plays racquetball three times a week for an hour. Or the patient with triple vessel disease who was scheduled for open-heart surgery but instead changed his diet and lifestyle and is now symptom-free.

In addition, I teach my patients many of the skills described in this book, meditation and positive affirmations as well as lifestyle and diet changes.

One of the most important ways to help enhance hope is to talk to the family. First speak hopefully to the family members themselves and encourage them to reflect positive attitudes around the patient. I emphasize to the family that their loved one is in a particularly fragile state of mind and needs their family's support. I tell them to take every opportunity to hug the patients and tell them how much they love them, how important they are to them. I speak as directly and honestly as I can, both to adult family members and to the children.

HOW TO EMPOWER PATIENTS

In addition to enlisting the healing force of hope, there is much we physicians can do to empower our patients and to encourage them to work toward their own recovery. The following techniques have great power to touch people's hearts and can induce profound changes in their behavior and lifestyle, leading to a higher level of health.

• Invite patients to share their experiences; share your own with them. After all, don't we doctors too have hearts? If, in the patient-physician relationship, experiences are not shared, the experiences and emotions the physician goes through will remain with him, often to the detriment of his own health.

I know that whenever I have revealed myself to a patient as a person, I have been rewarded with mutual support. There have been times when I have felt that a word of comfort was all I needed to continue my daily work. On several occasions that comfort came from patients who were very sick and had reason for much lower spirits than mine.

• Respect your patients' intelligence. If the patient thinks the physician knows everything and the physician thinks she herself knows everything, where is there any room for what the patient knows?

• Encourage patients to accept responsibility for their own health. This might seem too obvious to mention, but there is a big difference between just saying, "Exercise three to five times a week," and explaining why exercise is important to cardiovascular health and offering alternative ways for your patients to get that exercise.

• Create an active partnership for health with your patients. The American Heart Association encourages such partnerships, suggesting working with each patient on the following: a discussion of why coronary artery disease developed, a clarification of the risk factors, an emphasis on the importance of diet, exercise, and stress management. Try to make available a library of books, pamphlets, and videotapes on each subject.

• Promote patients' spiritual growth. For receptive patients, actively exploring the spiritual dimension can help in understanding the why of the disease as well as the how. Explain the intimate connection between mind and body to help evoke patients' own healing powers. Encourage your patients to look on disease as an opportunity for self-discovery and wellness.

PATIENT-PHYSICIAN COMMUNICATION INVENTORY

To assess your own abilities as a teacher, as well as a healer, explore the following questions. Answer as honestly as you can; then, as you read the discussion, think about ways you can improve your own patient-oriented practice. Remember that there are no right or wrong answers.

1. Do I give my patients enough opportunity to verbalize all their concerns?

Many physicians fail here, thinking that we have all the answers, or perhaps fearing to hear patients' legitimate concerns and fears. Learn to be quiet while your patients gather their thoughts; don't fear a few seconds' silence.

2. Am I impairing my patients' understanding by using technical language?

This is another example of the ways we distance ourselves

from our patients. Learn to use the more common words when appropriate. For example, say "heart attack" rather than "infarction."

3. Am I more interested in disease than in the patient?

In many cases, medical school taught us to look at "the gall-bladder" or "the hypertension" instead of Mr. Jones, father of three, or Ms. Abbot, the teacher with a shy smile. If we cannot be interested in the person who has the disease, we will not be able to work with that person toward a cure.

4. Am I limiting my remarks to "what is wrong," or do I stress "what is right" with my patients' health status?

This question is extremely important, because the element of hope can only build on the positive. Perhaps Mr. Smith eats well-marbled steak four times a week and is forty pounds overweight and has been unable to stop smoking. It looks bad, but at least encourage him for *trying* to stop smoking . . . perhaps he will succeed this time.

5. Do I project an image of infallibility, or do I come across as a human being?

We are taught, almost like priests, that a doctor must not fail, must not have feelings. In a sense this whole book refutes that notion. In my opinion, the more physicians can project their own humanity, the more patients will trust them and the stronger the healing partnership will become.

6. Do I empower my patients with knowledge and responsibility?

As I have mentioned, I created a conference room in my office, where I get together with my patients to discuss prevention of disease and wellness. I have assembled a wide library of books, pamphlets, and videotapes which patients are free to take home. By making these materials available, I feel I am empowering my patients with the tools they need to understand and begin to heal their own illnesses.

7. Do I resent my patients seeking another medical opinion?

This is similar to Question 5, in that it addresses the infallible image we physicians are supposed to project.

8. Do I avoid exploring my patients' emotional needs?

Again, I can't stress too strongly how important it is for physicians figuratively to drop their masks and interact with patients as fellow human beings. If you demonstrate your own humanity, you can't help but see and react to the humanity in your patients.

9. Do I enhance my patients' ability to recognize their own healing capacity?

The innate healing powers of the body have not been taught in medical school because they can't be quantified. As I said earlier, I believe we are on the cutting edge of a revolution in medicine, and as physicians we can help to lead that revolution. I urge you to read up on the literature of psychoneuroimmunology and share this information with your patients.

10. Do I honor my patients' decisions and judgment and give moral support when needed?

This is very important, even when a patient has made a decision you do not agree with, such as, for example, refusing surgery that you believe is necessary. Honor the patient's integrity and autonomy even if the patient does not accept your advice. You have done the best you can do; now allow the patient, as a fellow thinking and feeling being, to follow his or her own dictates.

A PATIENT'S WISH

The following meditation from a patient to his doctor sums up the fears as well as the hopes most of our patients have when confronted with the unknown territory of illness.

First of all, I want you to know how important it is for me to be understood. You know my diagnosis and you also have a plan for healing me. But you don't know me as a person. You don't know what the disease means to me, how I see myself now that I am sick. To me, how I experience my disease is more important than knowing exactly what disease I have. I need your help to deal with my feelings. I need your support when I feel sad and lonely. I need to be told that I can recover.

I need to be touched, to be hugged, to experience that you love me. I need hope and I need it from you, my doctor, whom I respect and admire. You can help me to perceive my sickness in a hopeful light; at the same time you can help me to stay in touch with reality. Please remember that, in addition to your knowledge, I need your presence. Don't just look at the chart and then leave me with only a word or two, alone in a frightening hospital room.

Understand that, most of all, I need hope. Hope that I will be able to leave this hospital, that I can regain at least some of my strength. Hope that I will be able to walk with my grandchild in the garden, that I will be able to fulfill my dreams. Hope that I can continue the life I led before this illness, that I will still be able to enjoy life with my friends and my family, even if not in exactly the same way. This heart attack that came so suddenly has changed me profoundly, has compelled me to think of myself and my future in a different way. I am no longer the same person. My values have changed, my love for family is closer to my heart than ever. My relationship with God, with the infinite, has changed, has become stronger. Please understand these changes and respect them.

As I will soon be starting the rehabilitation program, I need your support so that my heart will regain the strength I need to continue my life and my work. I appreciate it when you are willing to be present, to listen, and to hear my words without judgment. My heart is full of love and hope.

Bibliography

Benjamin, Harold H., with Richard Trubo. *From Victim to Victor: The Wellness Community Guide to Fighting for Recovery for Cancer Patients and Their Families*. Los Angeles: Jeremy P. Tarcher, 1987. A path to recovery for cancer patients.

Benson, Herbert. *The Relaxation Response*. New York: Avon Books, 1976. The application of Benson's relaxation technique, which has helped thousands of readers to cope with stress.

Borysenko, Joan. *Guilt Is the Teacher, Love Is the Lesson*. New York: Warner Books, 1991. Practical ways to deepen your self-knowledge and escalate to new spiritual heights of self-acceptance and self-love.

———. *Minding the Body, Mending the Mind*. Reading, MA: Addison-Wesley, 1987. A guide to self-growth through mastering stress and emotions.

Bradshaw, John. *Healing the Shame That Binds You*. Deerfield Beach, FL: Health Communications, 1988. How to gain the freedom to be and accept yourself.

Branden, Nathaniel. *Psychology of Self-esteem: A New Concept of Man's Psychological Nature*. New York: Bantam Books, 1969. A guide to understanding the origin of self-esteem and learning to develop it.

Charlesworth, Edward A., and Ronald G. Nathan. *Stress Management: A Comprehensive Guide to Wellness*. New York: Ballantine Books, 1990. An excellent guide to understanding and overcoming stress in your life.

Chopra, Deepak. *Unconditional Life: Mastering the Forces That Shape Personal Reality*. New York: Bantam Books, 1991. How to get in touch with the true self and experience holiness.

————. *Quantum Healing: Exploring the Frontiers of Mind/Body Medicine*. New York: Bantam Books, 1989. A profound guide to the body based on the premise that we become what we believe we are.

Cortis, Pia. "The Uncut Rose: A Pathway to the Unhindered Expression of Feelings." Unpublished manuscript.

Cousins, Norman. *Head First: The Biology of Hope*. New York: E. P. Dutton, 1989. How compassion and love are fundamental to the doctor-patient relationship.

————. *Anatomy of an Illness as Perceived by the Patient*. New York: Bantam Books, 1979. How to improve the patient-physician relationship, and the healing power of the mind over the body.

Dossey, Larry. *Space, Time, and Medicine*. Boulder and London: Shambhala, 1982. An explanation of the nature of time and how our perception of it affects our health, our lives, and illness.

Dyer, Wayne W. *Pulling Your Own Strings*. New York: Thomas Crowell, 1978. How to change your life by abandoning the victim role and taking responsibility.

Eliot, Robert S., and Dennis L. Breo. *Is It Worth Dying For? A Self-assessment Program to Make Stress Work for You, Not Against You*. New York: Bantam Books, 1984. The influence that stress has on our lives, including negative self-talks and how to change them.

Emerson, Ralph Waldo. *Self-reliance*. 1841. Mount Vernon, NY: Peter Pauper Press, 1967. A classic guide to inner peace.

Engel, Lewis, and Tom Ferguson. *Imaginary Crimes: Why We Punish Ourselves and How to Stop*. Boston: Houghton Mifflin, 1990. Key psychological problems and how to understand and forgive yourself.

Ferguson, Tom. *The No-Nag, No-Guilt, Do-It-Your-Own-Way Guide to Quitting Smoking*. New York: Ballantine Books, 1987. A comprehensive and informative guide to becoming a permanent nonsmoker.

Frank, Arthur W. *At the Will of the Body: Reflections on Illness*. Boston: Houghton Mifflin, 1991. The author's experience of illness, described in a profoundly human way illustrating what a patient-physician relationship can be.

Friedman, Meyer, and Ray H. Rosenman. *Type A Behavior and Your Heart*. New York: Fawcett, Crest, 1974. A guide to understanding Type A behavior and what to do about it.

Graedon, Joe, and Teresa Graedon. *Joe Graedon's the New People's Pharmacy*. New York: Bantam Books, 1985. A comprehensive and informative guide to prescription medicine.

Gibran, Kahlil. *The Treasured Writings of Kahlil Gibran*. Secaucus, NJ: Castle Books, 1985. Inspiring poems permeated by Eastern wisdom.

Hall, Manly P. *Healing: The Divine Art*. Los Angeles: Philosophical Research Society, 1972. A description of the theory and practice of metaphysical medicine.

Hay, Louise L. *You Can Heal Your Life*. Santa Monica: Hay House, 1985. Clear and practical suggestions and insights for a happy life.

Helmstetter, Shad. *What to Say When You Talk to Yourself*. New York: Pocket Books, 1986. How to discover and improve self-talks.

Holmes, Ernest. *The Science of Mind*. New York: Dodd, Mead, 1938. A fundamental book on mind healing through spiritual practice.

James, William. *The Varieties of Religious Experience*. 1902. New York: Mentor Books, 1958.

Jampolsky, Gerald G. *Love Is Letting Go of Fear*. Berkeley: Celestial Hearts, 1979. Twelve lessons for personal transformation and inner peace.

Jevne, Ronna Fay, and Alexander Levitan. *No Time for Nonsense: Self-help for the Seriously Ill*. San Diego: Lura Media, 1989. How to live fully with life-threatening illness.

Justice, Blair. *Who Gets Sick: Thinking and Health*. Houston: Peak Press, 1987. A lucid explanation of how mind and body interact.

Keyes, Ken, Jr. *The Methods Work If You Do*. Coos Bay, OR: Living Love Publications, 1980. A practical guide to personal growth and self-discovery.

Kübler-Ross, Elisabeth. *To Live Until We Say Good-bye*. Englewood Cliffs, NJ: Prentice-Hall, 1978. Lessons from dying people.

Lance, Kathryn. *Going to See Grassy Ella*. New York: Lothrop, Lee and Shepard, 1993. A fictional account of a child overcoming illness (for young readers).

Langer, Ellen J. *Mindfulness*. Reading, MA: Addison-Wesley, 1989. Illustration of the richness of life possible when we live in the present.

Laskow, Leonard. *Healing with Love: A Physician's Breakthrough Mind/Body Medical Guide for Healing Yourself and Others*. San Francisco: HarperSanFrancisco, 1992. Multiple exercises demonstrating the healing power of the breath; how to experience love as a healing force.

Levine, Stephen. *Healing into Life and Death*. New York: Doubleday, Anchor Books, 1987. A path to inner discovery.

Lynch, James J. *The Language of the Heart: The Human Body in Dialogue*. New York: Basic Books, 1985. Elucidates the hidden dialogue of the body and mind.

Mendelsohn, Robert S. *Confessions of a Medical Heretic*. New York: Warner Books, 1979. The problems of modern medicine and the importance of taking responsibility for your own health.

Mercer, Michael W. *How Winners Do It*. Winnetka, IL: Wellington Publishers, 1989. A practical guide for career success, very enriching and informative.

Missildine, W. Hugh. *Your Inner Child of the Past*. New York: Simon and Schuster, 1963. How to recognize and accept your inner child of the past.

Ornish, Dean. *Dr. Dean Ornish's Program for Reversing Heart Disease*. New York: Random House, 1990. Lucid explanations of how nutrition, exercise, and lifestyle changes may cause regression of coronary artery disease, proving also that inner peace is a pathway to wellness.

Pearsall, Paul. *Super Immunity*. New York: Fawcett, Gold Medal, 1987. How to control your immune system and promote higher levels of health.

Peck, M. Scott. *The Road Less Traveled: A New Psychology of Love, Traditional Values, and Spiritual Growth*. New York: Simon and Schuster, Touchstone, 1978. An inspiring guide to personal growth.

Rann, Michael C. *The Power of Commitment*. Chicago: Gamzo Advertising Consultants, 1982. An inspiring guide to success.

Risberg, Greg, and Virginia E. McCullough. *Touch: A Personal Workbook*. Oak Park, IL: Open Arms Press, 1989. Many insights on a basic human feeling, touch.

Schultz, John. *Writing from Start to Finish*. Portsmouth, NH: Boynton, 1990.

Shealy, C. Norman. *90 Days to Self Health*. New York: Dial Press, 1977. Practical pathways to wellness.

Siegel, Bernie S. *Peace, Love, and Healing*. New York: Harper and Row, 1989. With profound humanity and practical wisdom, demonstrates the path to self-healing.

Simon, Sidney B., and Suzanne Simon. *Forgiveness*. New York: Warner Books, Philip Lief Group, 1990. Illustrations of the power of forgiveness, leading to freedom and self-healing.

Simonton, Carl O., Stephanie Matthews-Simonton, and James L. Creghton. *Getting Well Again: A Step-by-Step, Self-help Guide to Overcoming Cancer for Patients and Their Families*. New York: Bantam Books, 1978. How to overcome cancer; the value of mental images.

Sinatra, Stephen T. *Lose to Win: A Cardiologist's Guide to Weight Loss and Nutritional Healing*. New York: Lincoln Bradley, 1992. How to achieve a healthy lifestyle with proper nutrition and self-love.

Tager, J. M., and Stephen Willard. *Transforming Stress into Power*. Chicago, IL: Great Performance, 1988. A practical guide to stress mastery.

Troward, Thomas. *The Edinburgh Lectures on Mental Science*. New York: Dodd, Mead, 1909. The relationship between spirit and matter, and how mental action affects material conditions.

Virshup, Bernard. *Coping in Medical School*. New York: W. W. Norton, 1985. A must for any medical student; an inspiring and practical guide for survival.

Widdowson, Rosalind. *The Joy of Yoga*. Garden City, NY: Doubleday, Dolphin, 1983. An illustrated guide to yoga.

White, Betty. *Pet Love: How Pets Take Care of Us*. New York: William Morrow, 1983. How to improve your life by loving a pet.

Whitehead, Carleton. *Creative Meditation*. New York: Dodd, Mead, 1975. How to attune yourself to the universal power and gain control of your life through creative meditation.

Williams, Redford. *The Trusting Heart: Great News About Type A Behavior*. New York: Times Books, 1989. The negative effects of hostility and anger, and how to improve health and life with a trusting heart.

Index

Invitation to Correspond with the Author

———————

Readers who are interested in learning more about the Exceptional Heart Patients Program, or who wish to share their own experiences in healing, are invited to write to the author at:

7605½ West North Avenue
River Forest, IL 60305

About the Author

BRUNO CORTIS, M.D., was born and raised in Sardinia, Italy.
He lives in River Forest, Illinois, with his wife, Pia, and
children, Veronica and Maximillian. Dr. Cortis is a practicing cardiologist. He was a professor at the University of
Turin, Italy, and an associate at the University of Illinois. He
is a board-certified internist and cardiologist, and a
pioneer in angioscopy and laser applications. He has
published over seventy articles, mostly on heart disease.
Dr. Cortis is the founder of the Exceptional Heart Patients
Program.